COOKING
AS
THERAPY

COOKING AS THERAPY

HOW TO IMPROVE MENTAL HEALTH THROUGH COOKING

Debra Borden, LCSW

alcove
press

Published in the United States by Alcove Press, an imprint of The Quick Brown Fox & Company LLC.

Alcove Press and its logo are trademarks of The Quick Brown Fox & Company LLC.

Library of Congress Catalog-in-Publication data available upon request.

ISBN (hardcover): 979-8-89242-203-1
ISBN (paperback): 979-8-89242-289-5
ISBN (ebook): 979-8-89242-204-8

Cover design by Holly Wales

Printed in the United States.

www.alcovepress.com

Alcove Press
34 West 27th St., 10th Floor
New York, NY 10001

First Edition: October 2025

The authorized representative in the EU for product safety and compliance is eucomply OÜPärnu mnt 139b-14, 11317 Tallinn, Estonia, hello@eucompliancepartner.com, +33757690241

10 9 8 7 6 5 4 3 2 1

This book is dedicated to the many clients and colleagues who had the courage and curiosity to entertain a revolutionary new therapy called cooking therapy. I hope being open to an alternative path has been as healing and helpful to you as following my passion has been to me. This extraordinary, experiential therapy is now a living, breathing, credible modality, and for any part I've played in that journey, I am truly grateful.

In memory

Of my two brothers, Mike and Bob, both gone way too soon. Though they were different, neither actually needed therapy, as each in his way was a living example of all we aspire to: friendship, kindness, laughter, family, and a spirit I can only hope to emulate. I'm so glad they're playing golf together once again, and I bet the balls go really far in heaven. RIP, brothers.

Contents

Introduction

Setting the Mental Health Table

Welcome to the world of cooking therapy! This revolutionary experiential therapy uses the processes in cooking, like heating, chopping, and layering, to help you gain self-awareness and insight as well as discover habits and behaviors that may be holding you back from optimum mental health. In the following pages, you'll learn how to work through stressful situations, improve self-esteem, find balance, create calm, stay positive, contemplate change, and more. You'll address and improve both emotional and situational challenges right in your own kitchen. And the best part—you need little or no culinary skills to get started. It's intriguing, isn't it?

Imagine turning meal prep into an opportunity for insight, understanding, or motivation to make a change. Whether you're preparing an appetizer, entrée, dessert, or even a sandwich, you can incorporate cooking therapy into the event. Not only will you learn about yourself, your patterns, and behaviors that you may want to change, but you'll have fun doing it. Who knew therapy could be seriously helpful without being terminally serious? Plus, at the end of every session you'll have a meal! As I often say, why not order up a side of self-esteem with that salmon? Especially important, you will learn the difference between cooking therapy and "just cooking."

Approach cooking therapy with an open mind and a willingness to explore a new method to change a behavior or pattern that is not serving you well. There are those who will tell you that "people don't change." I believe that's merely a trite sound bite for those who haven't yet figured out a way to do it. In fact, I think the opposite is true. What I *know* to be true is that often, people only change when it's too painful not to. To me, that essentially means that when you get to the point where the pain is too much to bear, there is also hope. It's about accepting that it's time to make a change, and with that resolve can come energy.

As a licensed clinical social worker (LCSW) and a pioneer in the field of cooking therapy, I've helped many individuals and families learn and incorporate the tools necessary to implement this revolutionary experiential therapy.

While I've been known as "The Sous Therapist™" for seven years, my journey to becoming the Sous Therapist™ could not have been predicted; there were no straight lines or specialty certifications. Cooking therapy evolved out of a need to develop a rapport with my clients and provide them with a portal they could access for improved wellness, lifestyle, and self-understanding. As my clients learned, so did I, and the mutual benefit began.

I began my clinical career as a certified school social worker, eventually becoming a licensed clinical social worker in New York and New Jersey and obtaining a certificate in play therapy. In conducting play therapy, I created a safe space for children to express themselves with the use of toys, games, stuffed animals, and figures. In my work with families, expanding my skills to work with young children was essential. I worked in schools and a women's wellness center and ran my private practice.

Later I became a community liaison for an adolescent and adult substance abuse and psychiatric outpatient facility and, finally, an adult substance abuse inpatient rehabilitation center.

As a traditional therapist I knew little about experiential therapies like art therapy, music therapy, or equine therapy. But many of the inpatient facilities were beginning to incorporate alternative and movement therapies, and I loved the idea of learning about them.

Over the course of time, I found that every time I was a participant, I was blown away. Equine therapy brought me to tears. I learned so much about myself as I tried to coax a beautiful horse into moving from one spot to another and failed to make it happen. I do not do well with failure or patience, and my perceived "failure" was actually a discovery about the behaviors I might want to change going forward. It took a concrete event to have that kind of an impact. In one session of sand play therapy, I learned more about the patterns in my family of origin than I had with any genogram I'd ever created.

As an LCSW, I've always worked with children and families. But it wasn't until I became an in-home therapist for the state of New Jersey that I discovered that cooking therapy might have a place in my clinical practice, especially with clients who had a hard time in the traditional "dyad" of talk therapy, where the therapist and client are one-on-one and making direct eye contact. An in-home therapist brings therapy to the individual or family in their home or in a space in the community such as a school, park, or even a restaurant. These clients may be limited by transportation or medical issues and would be unable to access therapy if it didn't come to them. As in all therapeutic breakthroughs, even mini ones, clarifying the root of an emotion can be a first step. For me, clarifying that cooking was an actual therapy was just that: the first step to helping others do the same.

I provided therapy for two hours a week. My more reticent clients, adolescents at home in the afternoons while their parents worked, often resented being "sent" to therapy at all and certainly had no stake in utilizing the "me time" that was costing them precious computer or phone time. Engaging them was a challenge, and even creating the all-important rapport that is necessary for progress was difficult. Two hours is a long time to talk to anyone, let alone a stranger that is being forced on you. So I often played games with them, took them for walks, or created other activities that would spark their interest and foster expression while at the same time promote an atmosphere of safety and connection.

One such game I invented was Feelings Jenga. Not only did the kids have to write a feeling on every block, but each time they removed a block from the tower, they would have to use it in a sentence. They often tried to get away with the simplest sentence, like "Sometimes I feel angry."

But I insisted they use the adjective in a deeper way. Eventually they would get to something like "Sometimes I feel angry when another kid disrespects me."

Progress. But how many games of Jenga can you play?

There is a popular therapy board game called the Ungame, and I used that as well. It contains a deck of cards with probing questions like "What freedom do you value the most?" and "How do you react when you feel frustrated?" Helpful, but the clients were mostly complicit only in the moment because they had no other choice. I did not feel movement, either during the session or when I returned the following week. There was no "stickiness" or mention of attempts to utilize any of the tools suggested.

Many of my families were carrying a lot of negative emotions as well as difficult life burdens, so I created the Backpack Game. First, similar to how we used the Jenga tiles, we searched for rocks outside, then wrote negative emotions on them, like *disappointment, resentment, jealousy, bitterness, anger, frustration, meanness*. The client would wear the backpack, and I would put all the rocks inside it and have them walk around for about five minutes. One by one, discussing the emotion, I'd remove them. The metaphor was how much lighter the backpack was and how much easier it was to handle your life, even in tough times, without those emotions weighing you down.

Still, it was very difficult to feel that I was helping anyone, and each week I seemed to be starting from square one. My adolescent clients seemed particularly uninterested in self-exploration or problem-solving, and I felt continually ineffectual. It's a tough way to feel week after week as a supposed helping professional.

In my role, I was allowed to take the clients out to a park or other public area, and the kids were always asking to go to Burger King. I remembered a time when I ran a group for high school girls at risk and observed the way bringing cookies could transform them from sullen and quiet to chatty and disclosing. It also occurred to me that my own memories of food were tied up with warmth and nourishment, and I thought perhaps that could go a long way toward developing rapport, which, as I said, is so important in the therapeutic relationship. As you may have guessed, we did not go to any fast-food restaurants. Instead, in the same vein as other experiential therapies in which doing is different than just verbalizing, I began to implement the new, legitimate, and fun modality of cooking therapy.

It was so successful it was scary.

Clients who couldn't identify even basic emotions were finding their voice in "shaping" raw meat into balls or "peeling" bitter rinds off a cucumber. One of those clients was twelve-year-old Nicole, who had been sent to therapy by the school and her family. Her dad had left the house and married his dental assistant, and they had a new baby. Her mom was bitter and angry and constantly bad-mouthing both her ex-husband and his new wife. Nicole was acting out in school and getting into fights, and her grades had dropped.

Nicole did not want to be herself anymore. In an almost textbook case of wanting her life to be different, she began refusing to answer to her own name. Instead, she assumed the name of a popular and beautiful character from a current movie. And yet she would not acknowledge that anything was wrong, responding to all my questions with "Everything's fine. I don't know why the school said that. It didn't happen."

After about four weeks of this, I shocked her by showing up with the ingredients to make turkey meatballs. My thinking was that if I changed up the setting so she didn't feel as much as if she were under the microscope, she might share a real feeling. I also thought it might be empowering for her to create something. After we added the egg and breadcrumbs to the ground turkey, I asked her to mix it up with her hands. I was thinking more as a cook at this point rather than a therapist. At first she thought it felt gross, which was actually the first emotion she'd ever shared, but then, as she mashed it all together, she got into it and began squeezing it all together and suddenly announced, "This is what I'd like to do to my new baby sister!"

Hmmm. Disturbing? Yes, but a real feeling. *Finally.* And because we could identify an actual feeling, this was a portal. Nicole began to talk about missing her dad and hating his new wife and baby. As so often happens, once Nicole felt comfortable sharing her feelings, they poured out. Suddenly, she began to mention a "friend" who was cutting herself and that she was worried about this "friend." It was then that I realized I'd only seen Nicole in long sleeves. Although I eventually referred Nicole to a higher level of care and a psychiatrist, I felt that I helped her. The recipe for shaping meatballs and meat loaf has gone through many evolutions and appears later in Chapter 6 as "Moderate Your Mood Meatloaf" (page 105).

My work with Nicole proved to me that I could incorporate cooking therapy into my practice, so I decided to employ it with my private clients.

I spend a lot of time making sure a recipe is perfect for each of my clients. First, I ask, will the recipe have appropriate processes to mirror positive steps or change? Next, what are the client's dietary or time constraints? Some recipes may have steps such as chopping for anger or simmering for patience, but the beauty of cooking therapy is that almost every recipe can be mined for the metaphors, mindfulness, and mastery that occurs when doing rather than talking. It's often easy to let the client choose.

This is why I created my 3M curriculum of Mindfulness, Metaphors, and Mastery for cooking therapy. I wanted to be able to quantify the benefits that were taking place in sessions, and I knew that a format would provide a clearer blueprint for clients and other mental health professionals. I knew that mindfulness, mastery, and metaphors were the three clinical keys and that, by consolidating them into a curriculum, it would be easier for all to understand and access. There are many examples of people who are using my 3M curriculum and finding therapeutic benefits through cooking without even knowing it and without a guide to help them delve even more deeply into feelings, habits, behaviors, and positive change. A November 2024 article in www.statista.com reports that cooking and baking are the favorite hobbies of Americans and come before reading, spending time with pets, video games, and outdoor activities. Why? Many respondents cited the therapeutic benefits of being in the kitchen. Tiffany McCauley of the Gracious Pantry explains that "cooking is therapeutic for me," relaying that the alone time and creativity are two of the reasons that cooking "soothes her soul" (Allen, n.d.). *Mindfulness*, anyone? Further in line with cooking therapy is the *mastery* she achieves when she says that not only does cooking provide comfort and stress relief, but "the entire process is … an escape with a delicious finale" (Allen, n.d.).

The BBC reports that cooking has been helpful to people with severe health diagnoses and terminal illness. One such patient is Maria Honeker, who claims cooking helped her through her "darkest days" and writes, "Cooking became a therapy for me. It was the one thing I could be in control of" (*Cooking Helped*, 2024). This element of control is present in cooking therapy as we choose ingredients, commit to being present and immersed in the process, and purposefully glean new and true notions of our feelings and desires.

At the other end of the spectrum is Camille Styles, editor and influencer at www.camillestyles.com, who writes that she turns cooking or meal prep into "a meditative practice" (Horstman, 2024). A champion of all things mindful, she advises readers to "focus on the task at hand and notice the colors and textures of the ingredients, sounds of cooking, and aromas filling the kitchen" (Horstman, 2024). Inadvertently, Camille has entered the mindfulness stage of cooking therapy as well as accessed the metaphors for noticing. No doubt the mastery in a completed dish or meal is evident as well.

Across the globe, people are discovering these three important elements of cooking therapy and the incredible benefits provided by using cooking as a therapeutic tool. An article in the *South China Morning Post* mirrors the elements of the 3M curriculum you'll find in the pages ahead. Nearly a third of respondents to a survey cited cooking as providing psychological relief. "Home cooking can have a positive impact on mental wellness as it engages both body and mind. I consider home cooking a holistic activity as it enhances a person's mental health in many different ways," said Mariana de Oliveira Dias, executive director of health and wellness at Sands China in Macau. "It reduces stress; allows creative freedom and self-expression by experimenting with different flavors, ingredients and techniques; provides a sense of accomplishment and pride," she added. "Seeing the end result is rewarding and boosts self-esteem; invites mindfulness, as you are fully present and engaged in the cooking process; and encourages you to slow down and savor each step of the process" ("How Cooking and Connecting," 2024).

It's important to incorporate mindfulness into every session to help clients disconnect from the bells, buzzers, whistles, and stressors of daily life. With metaphors, the substantive work of reflecting and evaluating patterns and behaviors can begin, and including a success into every session is optimal for self-esteem, confidence, and pride. We'll explore the 3M curriculum further in Part 1 of this book.

One example of the curriculum in action was with Nora, a wife and mother in her mid-thirties. Her husband's mood swings were volatile and unpredictable and had her on the verge of panic disorder. She was in therapy for the anxiety that was playing out at her job and with her children. She often had stomachaches and freely admitted she was short-tempered in the house. Nora was insightful enough to express that she was afraid she was troubleshooting her husband's moods rather than focusing on her own, ever.

For Nora, we chose to make cupcakes, and she expressed, "At least when the kids come home, I'll have something nice for them." I knew I could begin to use the metaphors of butter to soften, sugar to sweeten, flour as a kind of staff of life, and eggs to promote the "birth" of a new idea. But Nora was distracted and a bit hurried, and she accidentally added flour to the butter instead of sugar and frantically but unsuccessfully tried to scoop it out. Finally, she just gave up. Then she looked at me and said, "This is just like my marriage; no matter what I do, I can't save it."

This was something that came to her so clearly, without talking. She had never said those words aloud before, even though they had been "baking" inside. Now, seeing that metaphor and saying that statement aloud put her in a position of power where she could take the next steps, whatever they might be.

This is a great example of meeting the ultimate goal in therapy: a client improving. If a client is suddenly able to see a situation that has been entrenched, or stuck, and realize that by recognizing it they can now deal with it actively (or choose not to), then the power to change or improve now lies with them. The coveted *aha* or lightbulb moment is really a client saying, "You know, I never thought of it that way before." That's how insight happens. That's how growth happens. That's a door opening for change.

Nora and I eventually salvaged the recipe, and although the cupcakes were imperfect, we "doctored" them with frosting and sprinkles. Nora named this recipe "Confusion and Confession Cupcakes," and I knew I was onto something powerful.

Nora is just one of the many clients I've worked with whose lives have been transformed by cooking therapy. Cooking therapy is a guided journey to self-reflection through *how* you prepare a dish. I purposely prefer cooking therapy for mirroring real lives. I want it to be accessible and doable at every meal in every household. That means no matter your dietary needs or preferences, cooking therapy can be employed. If your household is vegan, kosher, dairy-free, or meatless, cooking therapy is for you. If you have allergies or food limitations, cooking therapy is for you. Whether you prefer baking, marinating, roasting, frying, slow-cooking, or even just pulling ingredients out of the fridge to concoct a meal, you can use cooking therapy.

Experiential Therapy Versus Talk Therapy

Cooking therapy is an experiential therapy, which is a therapy focused on doing and not just talking. There may be tools, activities, and games incorporated into a session.

In a typical talk therapy session, the therapist and client will meet in the therapist's office at a specific time on a specific day. The therapist will attempt to help the client express and explore a challenge or issue that brings the client into therapy. The therapist will listen, ask questions, elicit responses, and hopefully reflect back the client's words to understand and assure the client that they understand what the client is saying. Most important, success in therapy depends on rapport between the client and therapist as well as optimism, especially from the therapist, that the client can get well. The focus of traditional therapy is that rapport and conversation.

In experiential therapies such as art therapy, eye movement desensitization and reprocessing (EMDR), equine therapy, surf therapy, and cooking therapy, much less talk is used by the client and much more tangible or concrete activities are employed. The rapport comes from working side by side, or with the therapist as an activity guru, rather than simply with words. In art therapy, the client uses art materials for self-expression and exploration. In EMDR, the client is prompted to use rapid eye movements in different patterns to uncover internal distress, while in equine therapy, there is little or no conversation at all. By connecting to and handling horses, a client can learn confidence, learn how to bond, and uncover their own emotional setbacks, strengths, or even past trauma.

When I worked for a dual-diagnosis treatment facility in Florida, the patients were able to participate in surf therapy with trained surfing staff and clinicians. During therapy, patients spent a short amount of time in the shallow water near the beach learning to "surf." By surf, I don't mean to conjure up images of *Hawaii Five-0*. This essentially involved managing to get on the board, possibly kneeling or standing, and traveling even a tiny bit ... or not. Why was this a powerful and effective treatment? Some of the participants came to the beach with intense anxiety (drowning), fears (sharks), and irrational beliefs (imminent tsunami). Many had simply never learned to swim or had been in the ocean. And though the water was frightening to some, we also know it can be framed as nurturing and protective. It's womblike, after all. Helping a patient to feel lighter and "buoyant" was often a bonus.

Even a few steps into the water or a belly on the board was an accomplishment. Mastery involved a feeling and a result with legs—meaning many of us give so much mental space to our failures but no equal time to our successes! Learning to let our accomplishments fill us with insight and pride promotes mental health. As with cooking therapy, surfing was only part of the program, while the guided experience, the encouragement, the touch, reflection, and process rounded out the session.

There is even a therapy called "no-talk therapy" that is usually used with children. I've often used these techniques. The focus in no-talk therapy is on creating comfort through game play, pleasurable moments, and a variety of activities that purposely do not focus on talking. Martha Straus, in her book *No Talk Therapy for Children and Adolescents* (2023), details the way that tangible activities help children and adolescents to heal when conversation is limited or uncomfortable. She writes, "In No-talk Therapy, there is limited dialogue, but the conversations are rarely about problems and solutions. It is more about building kids' sense of competence, comfort in the therapy room, and control of their own behaviors."

Many other hands-on therapies are becoming widely used. Sand play, pet therapy, maze experience, and nature and hiking therapy are just some of the alternative modalities on the rise.

In cooking therapy, we incorporate the self-expression and exploration of art therapy, the distress tolerance and investigating of EMDR, the uncovering of patterns and habits and confidence building of equine therapy, the anxiety relief of surf therapy, the power of doing rather than talking of no-talk therapy, and the disconnect from technology featured in many of the other therapies—and we do it all at home, in your own kitchen. Unlike making an appointment with an art therapist or locating an equine facility, once you learn cooking therapy, you will be able to use it every single day with every single meal, if you choose. You can schedule it at your own time and for just the cost of your meal.

While these concrete or tangible therapies are never a *substitute* for talk therapy, they may enhance it. I've had many clients bring their cooking therapy experiences to traditional therapy and "serve" them as "food for thought" for both therapist and client.

People find their way to cooking therapy and other experiential therapies for a host of different reasons. Some are seeking to change, find balance, discover new ways to handle stress, improve self-esteem, or build better relationships. Others make their way into the kitchen after disappointment, loss, or grief. The attraction to nourishing our hearts and souls by nourishing our bodies in the kitchen may be subconscious but has been documented frequently. *Nourishment* is a powerful word, and for me, it slips easily from noun to verb. A recent article on TheStar.com tells the story of Sarimah Hania, who faced postpartum depression and found cooking to be her path to healing. Cooking as therapy became what Sarimah called "a powerful tool for self-expression, positive change, and a transformative journey" (Ihsan, 2024). I couldn't put it better. Cooking therapy creates movement and evolution and is fluid. If you are stuck, it can pull you up and out.

Your Road Map to Cooking Therapy

As you can see, cooking therapy is utilitarian and can be used in a wide range of settings and for so many emotions. As you read this book, you will learn to interpret and apply the lessons and guidelines in your own way based on your own assessments and decisions about what is happening in your own life. Therapy, any therapy, is for self-reflection and not to satisfy anyone except yourself. Often, clients find the therapeutic journey amorphous or ambiguous. Unlike with a physical illness, there is no pill prescribed or apparent treatment protocol. With cooking therapy, however, there is a clear construct to implement.

Ask yourself this:

- *What if* every time you prepared a meal, snack, or even a sandwich, you could also short-circuit the worry loop in your head, clarify a relationship issue, or explore a behavior pattern that is not "serving you" well?
- *What if* you could do it all in your own kitchen, at a time that works for you, and for no more than the price of the meal?

- *What if* your therapy did double duty? If along with that entrée of baked cod you could enjoy a side dish of clarity or a call to change?

With cooking therapy, you can...

- Sift flour.
- Add water.
- Stir together.

You might end up with bread. Or a sense of yourself. Probably both.

In the pages ahead, I will give you the tools and information you need to address common mental health issues with step-by-step instructions on how to be your own cooking therapist. Recipes can be customized for time, meal, and dietary needs/preferences as well as for couples, families, and groups.

In Part 1, you will learn about the science behind cooking therapy as a clinical therapeutic modality, how and why it works, and the many elements of other, more traditional therapies it incorporates. You'll learn about the many treatment centers, institutions, and organizations where cooking therapy is already being implemented, and you will begin to understand the three elements of my 3M curriculum—metaphor, mindfulness, and mastery—with examples of how I've used them in my practice and how you can too. Using my 3M curriculum, anyone can easily learn to master cooking therapy, either individually, as a couple, with colleagues in a group setting, or with family.

In addition to delving into the amazing power of this experiential therapy and the benefits of disconnecting from technology, we'll uncover the universal components in anxiety, depression, grief, and other common reasons clients come to therapy and learn how to use cooking therapy to address them.

Finally, I provide a handy list of cooking therapy processes and how they might inform your sessions in Part 2. Also in Part 2, we'll get cooking. I include specific and guided cooking therapy sessions based on emotional or mental health pursuits. In the first session in Chapter 6, we'll create calm. In session two, in Chapter 7, we'll develop self-confidence. In session three, in Chapter 8, we'll practice radical self-acceptance. In session four, in Chapter 9, we'll learn how to process sadness. We'll continue to build on these skills in session five, in Chapter 10, where we'll embrace the courage to change. And finally, in session six, in Chapter 11, we'll learn how to hear and be heard.

Under each topic will be three sessions based on the time you have to spend in total:

- **Fast Lane** will take you just five to ten minutes.
- **Easy Rider** will ask you to spend forty-five minutes to an hour.
- **Scenic Drive** will give you a leisurely and open-ended experience that may take an hour or up to several hours.

Then you'll have access to a list of over a hundred commonly used ingredients and suggestions on how to use them as cooking therapy components so that you can create a cooking therapy intervention for yourself anytime you access that ingredient.

Each session will have a specifically tailored recipe name to cement the goals and accomplishments learned in the sessions. At the end of each recipe, I'll provide you with a "to-go bag" that will include tips and metaphors from the session so that you can return at any time to remind yourself of all you've accomplished and cement the progress you made. Should you not feel like rereading or redoing an entire session, your to-go bag will serve as a handy reminder.

Now that you know a little bit about what cooking therapy is and how it might work for you, let's explore the clinical underpinnings that make this modality credible and universal. In the following chapters you'll learn about the science, the successes, and the surprises that await as you embark on your journey to wellness and positivity through cooking therapy.

PART 1

The Methods Behind the Magic

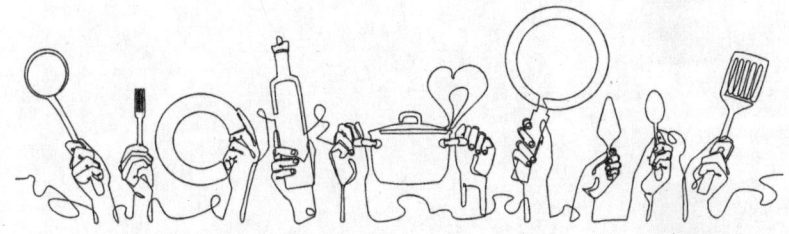

Chapter One

The Scientific Proof in the Pudding

In many ways, cooking therapy is like traditional therapy in that it's exploratory, self-reflective, and enlightening, but it's also different. When you're talking to someone, you're listening, speaking, and filtering thoughts in your brain, so awareness and change can take time. But cooking therapy is both visual and tangible and does not drive through the regular route of talk therapy. It takes you down a parallel path.

Think about the various pathways in your brain, through the amygdala, prefrontal cortex, or cerebellum. When you speak and listen, certain pathways light up. When you physically do a task, others are ignited. In simple terms, the left hemisphere of the brain, and particularly Broca's area, is activated during conversation and helps with processing ideas. From there, you can make decisions about how to act or behave. Conversely, when you perform a task, you activate a part of the prefrontal cortex, also involved with decision-making but more closely aligned with physical sensation and long-term memory.

As we begin to delve further into the science of cooking therapy, it will be helpful to understand the way that cooking therapy pulls from traditional and respected mental health disciplines while adding benefits germane to the cooking therapy process. The combination of traditional and respected psychiatric practices with credible experiential components will provide you with a robust and powerful mental health and wellness toolkit.

The Modalities of Cooking Therapy

Like other experiential therapies, cooking therapy is also a hands-on, tangible, clinical therapy that incorporates many modalities, including cognitive behavioral therapy, brief therapy, solution-focused therapy, gestalt therapy, and dialectical behavior therapy.

The foundation for cooking therapy is in cognitive behavioral therapy (CBT), a therapy founded by Aaron T. Beck in the 1960s. A key component in CBT is the recognition and reality checking of cognitive distortions. In other words, if you start out with the wrong thought, it is likely going to determine an erroneous feeling and produce an errant behavior. For example, if you tell yourself that people don't like you, chances are you will feel hurt or angry, and then you may interact with distance, or even a self-protective "unlikable" shell, and the pattern confirms the wrong thought and continues. When we challenge the first thought, ask how it came to be that you tell yourself you're unlikable, ask for evidence that makes it true, and discover that it may not be true, a new thought can replace the old one, a new and more positive feeling can be internalized, and new interactions can occur. Some other examples of cognitive distortions include "catastrophizing," which is always assuming the worst; "mind reading," assuming what others are thinking and feeling; and "black-and-white thinking," which allows only for two rigid thoughts or behaviors with no areas of gray in between.

The way we incorporate CBT into cooking therapy is seamless and effective. Actual food prep and processes mirror entrenched thoughts. A cooking therapist may ask, are we able to enjoy the cantaloupe if the shell is left on? The client recognizes the visual and is able to challenge a related thought that mirrors the unusable rind. The fact that the hard rind is unusable is reinforced and the benefit of removing it cemented. When the client removes the hard rind, they experience a completely new feeling (cool, orange, fresh). Instead of staring at an inaccessible melon, by peeling away the thought and replacing it with a sweeter or more palatable feeling, the behavior of pleasurable eating can ensue. The erroneous thought is noticed through mindfulness, the feeling is challenged or tweaked with metaphor, and a new habit or behavior is supported. To reiterate, the rind is the distortion, the melon the new and better feeling that results when the distortion is removed, and ability to "eat" the new feeling becomes a new behavior. Simply put, CBT states that when you change your thoughts, you change your feelings, and healthier behaviors follow. With cooking therapy, we do exactly that every time we prepare a meal or snack.

Cooking therapy is also the ultimate brief or solution-focused brief therapy (SFBT). In SFBT, the client identifies a targeted challenge, takes concrete steps to address it, and after a few sessions rates the benefits and/or success. SFBT is usually short term and can address singular situational events like test anxiety or larger subjects like future goals. The term *solution focused* means that successes, rather than problems, are highlighted and remembered. A therapist may use scripted questions like "Tell me about some of your accomplishments" or "Where are two places you've been the happiest?" to help the client develop their own strategies based on their own perceptions and past successes.

There are so many ways to use SFBT in cooking therapy. A recipe itself is a microcosm of a solution-focused task. In therapy, we identify an issue to address and hope to end up with a plan. In a recipe, our goal is to complete a short-term task by following the recipe and steps, and a dish is the result. Just as we might evaluate the success of a recipe for looks and taste, in a clinical cooking therapy session we evaluate the outcome by noting the insight gained or self-knowledge acquired.

In a cooking therapy session, any recipe, even one that's very short, can incorporate the tenets of SFBT. Perhaps a quick concoction of cinnamon toast might reflect taking an idea from soft to more formed (the toast). Then, a pat of butter, when spread, will hold the ideas. Next, the sprinkling of cinnamon and sugar can be employed as pros and cons. Finally, the warmth and melting, as well as the delicious smell, can mirror comfort in one's own creation and perhaps a plan.

Another famous and long-established psychological tool used in cooking therapy is gestalt therapy. In gestalt, clients are encouraged to examine their feelings by staying in the present rather than delving into past traumas or experiences. Clients are considered whole beings and are not defined by one event, situation, or diagnosis. Frederick Perls, the founder of gestalt therapy, said, "Awareness in itself is healing. Rather than sitting still and talking, you may be asked to actively participate in something like roleplay, you may assume the role of a person in your emotional circle and essentially play their part instead of your own" (Clarke, 2024). This is an effective tool for understanding how others see a situation and putting yourself "in their shoes." Guided imagery may be incorporated, where the client relaxes, closes their eyes, and is walked through an imaginary scenario filled with positive and relaxing associations, using them toward the goal of molding a happier mindset, reducing anxiety or pain, or even setting goals. Props are used to represent people and feelings and to help communication and understanding.

In my work with new clients who are less comfortable with insight and verbalization, I've used props to represent the weight of difficult situations as well as to incorporate metaphors. In cooking therapy, you might consider the entire meal a prop for understanding an issue that's hard to express solely with words. In gestalt therapy, it's believed that activities, often physical ones, create awareness, in a totally different way, and that through creative tasks a client can learn about themselves in a more whole way. Body language and even dreams are explored for their implications. A significant aspect of gestalt therapy is the therapist's role, which is seen as a partnership, with client and therapist as coworkers. The therapist will listen and interpret and encourage a client to stay in the present while examining feelings and emotions.

When seen through the gestalt lens, cooking therapy is an effective clinical tool. Being present is a constant in each cooking therapy session, and the partnership of client and therapist is obvious as they are literally working side by side. Each step in a cooking therapy session can help the client to explore current feelings and keep them from detouring into focusing on separate and singular traits, failures, or problems. Wholeness is represented in numerous ways, as so many recipes begin with separate ingredients that come together. The elements of gestalt are common when we focus on the end result rather than the parts. A session that's especially effective in a gestalt way is one where the client's hands mold parts into a whole, such as with a burger, meat loaf, or certain dessert concoctions that require rolling and shaping. In this way the client is encouraged to see the end result and totality rather than the spice of one or more ingredients. In this way, all three elements of cooking therapy are present: mindfulness for staying in the present, metaphors of wholeness rather than parts, and finally, mastery at recognizing one's achievement as a totality.

Finally, many of the tenets of dialectical behavior therapy (DBT) can be accessed with cooking therapy. DBT is an involved and multistep clinical modality that addresses four core skills: mindfulness, emotional regulation, distress tolerance, and interpersonal effectiveness. The metaphors in cooking therapy are precisely tailored to mirror the basics of DBT skills.

Here are a few examples. Mindfulness emerges in noticing senses such as sight, touch, and smell. We may simply stare at a bowl of fruit or breathe in the smell of cookies baking or notice the sound of chicken sizzling or the feel of kneading raw dough. Emotional regulation is targeted with tasks such as "bringing to a simmer" or "turning down the heat." It's incredibly impactful to actively engage in this process while comparing it to lowering internal pressure or reactions. Distress tolerance occurs in performing steps that are more difficult or unfamiliar, perhaps something as simple as cracking eggs without getting shells in the batter or whipping cream just enough to form soft peaks or even bringing candy to the hard-crack stage, which is both an impactful visual and an impactful phrase. We'll explore interpersonal effectiveness in session six, Chapter 11.

Performing the cooking therapy sessions in this book and becoming comfortable with the processes involved will make it easy for you to incorporate the features of any or all of the therapies I've mentioned. Now that you know the basic underpinnings of CBT, SFBT, gestalt therapy, and DBT, I will guide you to becoming skilled at recognizing and implementing the elements of any therapy that resonates with you both in cooking therapy sessions and as you live your life.

Cooking Therapy Is Fun

Cooking therapy has serious benefits and is also fun. Recent studies on laughter reflect the old tenet *Laughter is the best medicine*. The Mayo Clinic reports that there are both short- and long-term benefits from laughter. In the short term, laughter can stimulate many organs. "Laughter enhances your intake of oxygen-rich air, stimulates your heart, lungs and muscles, and increases the endorphins that are released by your brain. It can activate and relieve your stress response. A rollicking laugh fires up and then cools down your stress response, and it can increase and then decrease your heart rate and blood pressure. The result? A good, relaxed feeling" (Mayo Clinic Staff, 2023). Laughter also soothes tension by "stimulating circulation and aiding muscle relaxation, both of which can help reduce some of the physical symptoms of stress" (Mayo Clinic Staff, 2023).

Just as laughter can boost your mood, it can enhance a cooking therapy session. First, when we laugh, we relax. For many people, therapy of any kind is stressful, and laughter can be a natural and unstructured exercise in relaxation so that you can be truly present as you engage in a session. Next, there is humor to be found even in many of the serious cooking therapy tasks. For example, creating clouds of flour by clapping your hands together may spark a commitment to "creating clarity" and letting the dust fall, but it's also rather silly, and it's okay to enjoy getting clear and also having fun. Another fun part of cooking therapy can be naming the recipes.

Years ago, I created a cooking therapy video for a cooking show competition, and I decided to target divorced women whose husbands had had extramarital affairs. For fun, I suggested that we make sausage and peppers and use a huge butcher knife to chop those sausages into pieces. Of course, we then threw them into the pan with sliced potatoes and peppers and sizzled them till they were quite burnt. I jokingly named the recipe Lorena Bobbitt Bangers and Mash. (Lorena Bobbitt is famous for cutting off her cheating husband's private parts while he slept.) I didn't win the competition, but I did learn that many of us are craving more smiles and moments of silliness.

While embarking on your own cooking therapy journey, feel free to create your own funny and even irreverent sessions. There are many ways to exorcise negative feelings and still have laughter and fun. In fact, I'd suggest that many ingrained emotional irritations could be replaced and reframed with a funny new take in a cooking therapy session.

Short-term benefits and moments of fun are great, but many of us are concerned with weighty, long-term issues such as illness progression and other problems as we age. Years ago, the idea of healing cancer through laughing was radical and even thought unprofessional by some. Today, so many books exist that tout the effects of laughter on improving life expectancy, or at least attitude, which has been shown to have a direct correlation with health. Additionally reported by the Mayo Clinic is that laughter can boost your immune system. "Negative thoughts manifest into chemical reactions that can affect your body by bringing more stress into your system and decreasing your immunity. By contrast, positive thoughts can actually release neuropeptides that help fight stress and potentially more-serious illnesses" (Mayo Clinic Staff, 2023). It's been shown that laughter reduces pain and improves mood. "Laughter may ease pain by causing the body to produce its own natural painkillers, increase personal satisfaction and make it easier to cope with difficult situations. It also helps you connect with other people" (Mayo Clinic Staff, 2023).

Think about the power of this concept and how a cooking therapy session might affect someone who is dealing with an illness or injury. Imagine them being able to incorporate fun into an easygoing activity that provides self-insight but with no pressure. Those facing chronic or sudden illness may battle depression. Mood disorders, such as SAD (seasonal affective disorder), often create fatigue and lack of interest in outside activities. Cooking therapy can boost a person's resolve to be happier.

Benefits of Cooking Therapy

Cooking therapy is the perfect activity to combat shame, anxiety, and even indecision. Let's look at some of the tremendous benefits of this experiential therapy.

How the Three M's Make a Difference

With *mindfulness* comes the ability to be still with oneself, a difficult task for many. Being still can become a muscle memory and helps with every aspect of honest evaluation and decision-making. Often, I ask clients to simply smell a dish cooking, without talking. Many become uncomfortable after just thirty seconds. However, when prompted to continue in that semi-meditative state, they become more and more comfortable turning down the default response to move and can be more reflective, calm, and self-explorative.

A prominent example of this can be seen at the Kripalu Center for Yoga & Health, an educational mindfulness nonprofit. At Kripalu, among other benefits of accessing the mind-body connection, "the tool of mindfulness has been touted to be more helpful than talk therapy for depression." Mindfulness can trigger present-moment pathways and helps us disengage from negative self-talk and self-defeating pathways.

With *metaphors*, a client can explore their behaviors, cemented thoughts, and triggers in a safe way. For example, one of my families' sons had been diagnosed with oppositional defiant disorder (ODD). This family had been in the system for years, had seen multiple therapists and psychiatrists, and their son, James, now eleven, had been on a variety of medications since the age of five. Not only was there little improvement in James's behaviors, but he was getting bigger and stronger and his acting out had had physical consequences, including a wall being punched in and a back door torn half off the hinge. James's episodes of anger and acting out were increasing in school, and he was in a special education class, despite being very bright, due to his emotional dysregulation.

After only fifteen minutes I could sense that the mom's sadness, the dad's frustration, and James's inattention would benefit from something novel. If nothing else, I sensed it would shake things up. When I suggested cooking therapy, they all looked at me like I was crazy, but I also sensed a tiny curiosity and maybe relief that the next session would not be a rinse-and-repeat of all the previous ones. Since positive family time was in short supply, I decided that we'd make something the family could share for dinner after I left. After assessing for likes and dislikes, I suggested personal pizzas. I brought the dough, sauce, and shredded cheese and asked the family to have one or two other toppings, such as mushrooms or onions, available. During the session, we talked about the dough being the base of who we are and how we all start out the same, and how the sauce being spread can cover our traits or dreams or goals. But then we also discussed how the sauce could be a base, not a cover, for new ways to add those traits or dreams or goals back.

Each person added a topping or two and named something they wanted for themselves. When James announced that he wanted "everyone to leave me alone," sprinkling cheese provided a great portal to ask him how we could accomplish that. With each sprinkle, I asked him a way he could get his parents off his back. Eventually, we went from "I don't know" to a few key behaviors, such as tone of voice and "responding, not reacting."

It created a great dialogue for this family and added a new and fun way to interact. It also interrupted their pattern of feeling like the needy, broken family.

When it comes to *mastery*, if I could script a success into every client's life, that might have even more benefit than the actual therapy. Some clients in therapy can feel damaged or hopeless. Committing to and participating in a cooking therapy session from beginning to end is an accomplishment, no matter how the dish turns out. When I'm feeling low, I do it myself, if only with store-bought foods from the fridge. I may scoop some salad into a bowl, being mindful of the different colors and textures, checking in with myself about the various pieces of my life and how they're going. Then I might sprinkle a little Parmesan cheese, asking myself what parts of my life need more attention, and finally add dressing while reminding myself to add flavor at least once in my day. It feels so great to accomplish that mini session. Hopefully I follow through, but even if I don't, I've set my intent, just by performing a sliver of cooking therapy, and that is a success.

During cooking therapy, a participant is actively seeking thoughtful examination and self-reflection, and that is the component that also engages all the senses. In this way, a session has moments that mirror what positive psychologists call "the flow," a state where you're fully absorbed, goals are clear, and satisfaction is high. This will be especially true when you learn the skills to do cooking therapy by yourself.

Cooking Therapy vs. Cooking

It's important to understand the difference between cooking therapy and "just cooking," although eventually you'll be able to incorporate cooking therapy into just about everything you prepare in the kitchen if you choose.

Cooking therapy is purposeful and targeted. A baking pie may smell wonderful, but without the direction for self-reflection, metaphor, and evaluation, it's just baking, and simply a different, possibly rewarding, but not clinically credible event. Think of it like this: You're in the gym and you may know how to walk on an elliptical machine or treadmill, but you've never tried weight training. If you simply get on the equipment or lift the free weights, you may get some benefit, but you basically have no guidance as to form or reps and possibly no clue what muscles you are targeting. There is even a chance you might do things the wrong way. You need a trainer, at least at first, to guide you through the process. This is exactly why it's important to distinguish between cooking and cooking therapy. I want to make sure you get the full, clinical benefit of cooking therapy as well as the tangential infusions of warmth, memory, and joy.

Triggering That *Aha* Moment

Studies of experiential therapies have shown that they can activate different parts of the brain than talk therapy does. Some evidence suggests that these therapies are especially effective in reducing feelings of hopelessness and negative thoughts. Many clients in therapy feel stagnant. It's not unusual to hear clients complain, "I have nothing new to talk about." In fact, studies show that boredom and feelings of lack of substantial progress are two of the reasons clients leave therapy. In cooking therapy, emotional processing, creativity, and reflection are all contributors to a client's understanding of themselves.

Because cooking therapy is experiential and guided, the processes involved in preparing a recipe or meal will trigger thoughts and *aha* moments in a different way than traditional therapy. As mentioned before, though never a substitute for talk therapy, what is learned in a session can often support or enhance work done in a more typical session. In fact, many therapists are interested in learning from their clients who have experienced new or different thoughts in alternative sessions; this can inform both the clinician and the work. If therapy has "stalled" or is repetitive, experiential therapy can open a fresh portal for both therapist and client. Both in session and out, experiential therapies are considered evidence based and effective for treating a variety of mental health conditions, including anxiety, depression, family conflict, trauma, and addiction.

A review article in the journal *Health Education & Behavior* found that "cooking seemed to increase self-esteem and improved psychological well-being; it also appeared to decrease anxiety and agitation in a variety of people, including burn victims and those with dementia. Experts hypothesize that the activity can be soothing for several reasons. For one, it engages several senses, making it quite immersive" (Farmer et al., 2018).

Jamie Friedlander wrote an article for the *Washington Post* about her own journey to using cooking to quell anxiety. She quotes clinical psychologist Trevor Shraufnagel, associate director of the Anxiety Disorders Clinics at UCLA: "Because of this sensory engagement, cooking can be a form of *mindfulness*. Mindfulness often entails trying to focus on one thing in the moment—maintaining one's attention on a single sensory stimulus, such as the sound of oil crackling, the taste of a sauce, the smell of something baking or the sensation of one's breath. Several studies suggest mindfulness-based practices can play a role in the treatment of anxiety. Another possible explanation for why cooking may ease the symptoms of anxiety is that it can help people to feel both accomplished and in control" (Friedlander, 2020).

A study done by the National Library of Medicine (NLM) and National Institutes of Health (NIH) culled the clinical literature from approximately 2007 to 2017 for psychosocial benefits of cooking and found that inpatient and community-based cooking interventions yielded positive influences on proactive socialization, self-esteem, quality of life, and affect. In simple terms, it was an antidote to isolation, feelings of failure and/or gloom, and boredom.

Two research studies from the NLM and NIH study reported changes in confidence and/or self-esteem because of participation in structured cooking interventions. Generally, a small sample of mental health patients that participated in unit-based baking classes reported improved self-esteem, primarily because of increased concentration, coordination, and confidence. Participants reported that producing a product they could keep or give away to others was additionally beneficial and rewarding. The "increased concentration" mentioned in this study is my version of mindfulness. These days we are all pulled in so many directions that just being still is an achievement. Add in the metaphors for confidence and success and you have a perfect recipe for growth.

Years ago, I facilitated a weekly activity support group for the siblings of IDD (intellectual development disorder) clients who were living in group homes. These siblings were experiencing unique emotional journeys, but each was adjusting to having a sister or brother with major intellectual and/or physical challenges. Ages ranging from five to twelve meant that the support group had to have an activity that was fun and appropriate for a wide age range; cookie decorating was a huge success. In these sessions, even young children could integrate the sense that they were not the only ones who had a different family construct. Even more, the fun activity could be seen as a type of reward, suggesting that different is not necessarily bad. During the activity, children would talk freely while decorating their cookies. Sometimes they'd say things like "My sister likes pink, but she couldn't do this." It wasn't exactly cooking therapy, but many of the components were there: mindfulness as they focused on a task, metaphors of creating and being something special, and mastery at their creative concoctions. With young children, it's the foundations of cooking therapy that are the goal rather than deep, substantive revelations.

Out and About With Cooking Therapy

Cooking therapy rooms and classes are on the rise in schools, institutions, and organizations. Here are just a few examples of the settings where you can find cooking therapy and why they are impactful and successful:

- In June 2024, the Autism Behavioral Center (ABC) added cooking therapy to their programs. They affirm that "learning to cook can build confidence, foster independence, and create a sense of accomplishment."

- In March 2024, the Northeast Georgia Health System in Gainesville, Georgia, partnered with Lifepoint Rehabilitation to provide an entire therapy suite incorporating a cooking therapy room. Imagine rehabilitating from a traumatic brain injury or stroke and being able to use all your senses, especially if verbal or thought processes are compromised.

- At Beachside Rehab in Florida, a rehabilitation center for substance abuse, culinary healing nourishes "both body and mind." There, it's been noted that cooking can become "a therapeutic cornerstone" in the recovery process (LaGuardia, 2024).

- At Cirque Lodge, a treatment center for trauma as well as addiction, cooking therapy is recognized as "a method that integrates the art of cooking with traditional therapeutic practices in order to assist individuals in their journey toward recovery."

- Recovery Centers of America, Alta Loma Transformational Services/Lionrock in Texas, Newport Academy, and multiple senior living centers such as TerraBella, Auburn Hill, and Signal Mountain are just a few of the many organizations beginning to recognize the role of food and cooking in our emotional lives. For seniors, it's an activity that can be done independently or in a group setting. With loneliness and isolation becoming one of the major contributors to depression and even suicide in the elderly, an activity that creates warmth, engagement, and achievement is so powerful.

- The Chicago School, a leading nonprofit university, has set out to create their own curriculum around cooking therapy. Dr. Michael Kocet, PhD, chair of the Counselor Education Department, began this project more than seven years ago.

No matter your age or situation, it's no wonder that food and preparing meals "stirs up" so much memory and feeling. You needn't be coping with an incident, addiction, loss, or trauma to benefit. Cooking therapy works for those of us just trying to get through the day. The term *comfort food* first appeared in a 1966 article in the *Palm Beach Post* newspaper. It's been noted that comfort foods cause the release of dopamine, creating pleasure, possibly due to the high caloric composition. But comfort food can also bring back fond memories of childhood or home cooking and is often eaten when feeling overwhelmed or under duress. I believe that's the underlying explanation when people say "Cooking is my therapy" and love to cook. They find it comforting or relaxing and can "lose themselves in the activity." At the foundation of cooking therapy is a sensory experience. This immersion is formidable. And yet the clinical experience occurs when the experience is guided and the metaphors are examined for parallels to real life.

As you can see, cooking therapy incorporates many therapeutic modalities and is being incorporated into many institutions and programs. Cooking therapy can be appropriately implemented to address a variety of emotional and situational challenges, from anxiety and depression to indecision and life transitions, and is appropriate for all ages, from very young children to seniors. The sessions can create self-awareness, highlight cemented and unhelpful self-talk and negative patterns, and boost mood, inspiring laughter and fun that can revive a stagnant therapeutic journey. Mindfulness, metaphors, and mastery are all important components of cooking therapy that distinguish it from "just cooking," and this 3M curriculum will be explained and explored in detail in the chapter ahead.

Chapter Two

Lighting the Cooking Therapy Fire With the 3M Curriculum

There's an expression that "sports are a metaphor for life." This expression asks us to consider whether people's behaviors and emotions while playing certain games are fair, competitive, angry, cheerful, etc. Presumably you can learn a lot about people and how they behave in life from the way they behave on the field or court.

The same can be said about cooking therapy, but in an even deeper way. Cooking therapy is diagnostic, meaning performing tasks can mirror one's behaviors in life, leading to a revelation or a diagnosis. For example, are you reluctant to try something new or do the work? Do you begin with confidence or, conversely, the sense that you won't be able to accomplish a task? Do you feel overwhelmed and contemplate taking shortcuts? Do you immediately ask for help, or are you confident and excited to begin?

If you find yourself reluctant or hesitant, this shouldn't cause you anxiety or concern. Most of us are a bit tentative when beginning something new and unfamiliar. Instead, let's use the next chapter as a beginning exercise in getting in touch with our feelings, which is the first step toward self-understanding. As always, identifying reluctance or hesitation or even impulsivity is often a picture window to go through for discussion and revelation. As we further explore the three foundational principles of the 3M curriculum, it will become easier and easier to apply them to guided and self-study sessions, and in no time they will become second nature every time you choose to turn any meal prep into a cooking therapy intervention.

Let's break down how the 3M curriculum works.

Mindfulness

This is the very first step in a cooking therapy session. Unlike meditation, mindfulness in cooking therapy is an active step, less about breathing and more about being present as you perform each task.

First, you'll be mindful of your feelings before you begin. When you wash your hands, you'll be focusing on clearing out negativity and starting a fresh experience. Each step will be purposeful. Although there are moments when it's important to pause to take in sights, smells, sounds, and thoughts, for the most part you'll be mindful while *doing*. In meditation, you might be focused on breathing and being still. In cooking therapy, we'll concentrate on multiple observations. You'll pause to cement a feeling or thought so it sticks. You'll notice how you feel when you listen to the sounds of water boiling or a processer grinding or sausages sizzling. You'll observe the way a bowl of berries looks or a pot of soup smells, or how a batter swirls and how you feel as you stir, and you'll immerse yourself in noticing rather than "mindlessly" doing. Without bells and buzzers to distract you, you'll be able to be quiet with yourself while observing. And when you do, you'll be surprised to learn how calming and fulfilling it is to notice how wonderful noticing makes you feel.

One couple wrote me to tell me that they'd practiced my "Sesame Newdles" recipe on their own and experienced a particularly powerful and unexpected moment. When they "plunged the hot noodles into the ice bath," they reported that it was such a strong and concrete metaphor for letting the steam of anger go that they both used it the next time they felt themselves heating up for an argument. They actually say "Ice bath" out loud. It has become a colloquial verbal trigger, and a relationship helper, for each to say to the other if things are getting too hot.

I promise you will develop your own powerful moments of mindfulness that will stick with you long after the sessions are over.

Metaphors

If mindfulness is the quiet piece in cooking therapy, then metaphors are the loud, noisy alarm bells, not in an audible way but for their power. While each component of the 3M curriculum is weighty, it's the metaphors that clients often remember the most, both within the session steps and days or weeks after. In fact, I recently received an email from a client who participated in a women's weekend retreat with me, and she jokingly stated, "Thanks a lot Debra! Now I can't even make a sandwich without thinking of the layers in my life!"

The metaphors will stay with you long after the session. They begin with *gathering ingredients* (personality traits or expectations), *washing hands* (removing old muddy thoughts), and, if applicable, *preheating the oven* (heat being a catalyst for change). After that, all the cooking processes are fair game to mine for metaphors. Common ones include *peel away, uncover softness, chill till firm, let sit, watch rise, bring to a simmer, sift through, stir gently, let come together, sprinkle in, and don't over-beat.* One of my favorite cooking metaphors comes from a common instruction when preparing scallops. Once the scallops are browning in a pan, the instruction is "Don't harass the scallops." How great is that to cement the idea that sometimes you have to leave someone or some discussion alone.

That said, it's not just about teasing out the metaphors but also using them to examine behaviors, communication strategies, self-talk, relationships, and habits. Metaphors shine a light on feelings that may be errant, negative habits you may have cemented, and behaviors that result. The beauty of the metaphors is in the way each reader will assess their own patterns and decide if they are positive or negative, helpful, or destructive. That's a shared journey between the therapist, guiding you through the process, and you, applying them to your own life. Then, once you learn the skills from *Cooking as Therapy,* I hope you will have the courage to try to be your own culinary therapist. It's hard to look at yourself with just words, but metaphors in cooking lead to questions that are clear and strong. *Is there something bitter encasing you? Do you have a "secret pit" inside? How long does it take for you to boil? What might you incorporate to make the dish sweeter?*

Additionally, certain processes are more suited to different feelings. For example, chopping lends itself to reducing large problems into manageable parts, a goal of any therapy, while reduction can solidify a loose plan into an intense resolve. Sifting can "get the hard parts out," and blending has multiple uses. These are just a few examples.

Metaphors also model evolution. A recipe unfolds, steps ensue, and a dish becomes, and that's a metaphor for therapy itself.

Finally, the metaphors live in the names of the recipes, which always reflect the session. From "There's the Rub Rub," a spice blend, to "Sheet Happens" for sheet pan chicken, you will remember the lessons learned simply by recalling the recipe name.

One of my favorite sessions was sparked by an event I did for Sub Zero Group at the San Diego Food + Wine Festival, where I had the honor of copresenting with Katie Lee Biegel of the Food Network. I have to say, it was a lovefest, not only for Katie and me but also for the sheer number of people who stopped by our booth for kitchen therapy. The idea of self-help through cooking is one that many people immediately get. Katie and I focused on the ease of being in the kitchen with no pressure from friends, family, or even uncooperative appliances. One of the recipes she sent to me following the show was her favorite mashed potato recipe, which she credits to Jeff Mauro, called "The Creamiest, Butteriest, Tastiest Mashed Potatoes Ever." She was most certainly spot-on about the recipe, but I was so delighted with the many metaphors in the steps, such as drain, blend, grease, pour, and melt, that I had even more fun customizing it for a virtual cooking therapy session and renaming it "The Healingest, Definiest, Restoringest Mashed Potatoes Ever!" The only downside? My client told me her husband liked the potatoes so much he told her to stay in therapy forever!

Mastery

Everyone who participates in therapy is looking to feel better about something. Successes, even small ones, have the ability to empower, enrich, and build the kind of confidence that translates to healthy choices, improved self-esteem, and better emotional health. People who are proud, bloom. This applies to clients in outpatient therapy as well as those whose deeper issues benefit from residential or inpatient treatment. Many individuals in treatment can feel especially low and as if they are "less than" or have failed. Those struggling with addiction, for example, can have a history of others trying to help them and a sense of continuing to let people down. Consequently, one of the reasons many substance abuse facilities enlist their residents in volunteering is for the feeling of being helpful to others. Imagine how it feels to give when you've always been the person who takes. Imagine years of thinking of yourself as weak and suddenly being strong enough and worthy enough to help another. This is mastery in action. It can be life-changing.

For these reasons, the sense of accomplishment that can be obtained in a cooking therapy session is remarkable. In fact, it's an accomplishment that can be obtained daily, and that's even more significant.

During a cooking therapy session, though scripted, there will also be ample opportunity for choice and creativity. It's been noted that creativity itself contributes to feelings of independence and joy that can translate into a better mood. One study mentioned in the online blog *The Conversation* focuses on the benefits of creativity on the brain. They report that "every single session of real and honest self-expression can improve self-confidence, and reduce feelings of stress, anxiety and burnout because creativity activates reward pathways in the brain."

Completing a session results in an infusion of pride that can generalize from the session into a client's life. In this way, cooking therapy can create portals and open channels where growth and openness can spread like positive tree roots, taking hold in many ways and in many areas.

Kyle, age sixteen, was referred to me by his school's counselor. His parents reported that Kyle was becoming increasingly morose and isolated, especially at home, and uninterested in any family time, including with his younger brother, Ben, eleven, with whom he had always been close. Though Kyle still maintained some friendships, he'd stopped bringing his friends home and had given up basketball, which he previously enjoyed. His mom reported that the basketball games had been a family event and that they "hadn't missed a game, home or away." These changes in events and Kyle's demeanor had both parents worried.

Kyle understood why his parents were concerned and didn't dispute their report but couldn't offer any concrete explanations for the change. He stated that he was just "bored" with basketball, he had "nothing in common" with his little brother right now, and his "isolating" was "just what normal kids do." I wasn't convinced. Kyle was spending an awful lot of time on social media, like most teens, but dropping out of basketball was concerning. His room was covered with elementary school trophies and posters of Kobe Bryant and Michael Jordan. Also, I wondered about the involvement of his parents. Could they be overly involved and having difficulty with a teen beginning to individuate? It took three sessions alone with Kyle for me to decide that it might be helpful to have a family cooking therapy session. First, I wanted to see how the family interacted, but I also planned to have a session that involved choices.

Because we had only an hour, I decided we'd make ice cream sundaes with a variety of toppings. I told them the session would be called "Connections Concoctions." Kyle thought it was "kinda stupid" but was compliant. Little brother Ben watched his brother for his reaction and parroted, "Yeah, stupid." I felt the parents were being cautious not to seem too invested, and I understood. Often with teens, when your parents like something, that's reason enough not to! I did encourage creativity and asked everyone to try a topping or flavor they might not ordinarily use. I thought this was a great metaphor for entertaining newness and change.

The revealing part of the session did not come during the session itself. The family enjoyed exploring metaphors about the coolness of ice cream being a good base for identifying something cool about the "base" of who they are, and even Ben joined in. They were happy to "top" or "sprinkle" categories of things they enjoyed or for which they were grateful. There was no earth-shattering breakthrough, but it was fun. Which isn't a bad thing. Afterward, we processed, and it led to a healthy discussion of how communication helps with learning about yourself and sharing that information with others. Kyle stated that he needed to feel less "smothered" (brought out by chocolate syrup) and his parents and brother needed to still feel "loved" (the swirling and covering with whipped cream). Again, nothing monumental, but still positive.

What happened next is a testament to giving therapy a chance to "marinate and percolate" in the days or weeks following a session. When I arrived the following week to meet with Kyle, his mom pulled me aside to tell me that something interesting had happened with his dad. He'd been feeling underappreciated at work and started thinking about the ice cream toppings. The idea of creating new choices and ideas prompted him to talk to his boss, and the result was an additional role at the company that he relished. Talk about a bonus, in every way.

With cooking therapy, you can expect the unexpected.

I promise you that every cooking therapy session will incorporate mastery. You may be wondering how that can happen just by making a bowl of cereal or a baked potato. The cooking therapy tools you learn can turn even a small moment into a large success because of the mindset, commitment, and involvement in the therapeutic journey. You will see that bowl of cereal or baked potato in a new way, and it will change the way you think and feel.

In addition, there will never be a failure, even if a recipe doesn't turn out as you expected or "just like the picture." No matter the outcome, the important result is that you were there, focused, and present. Remember, the important part is showing up.

There's an expression among clinicians: *The therapy begins with the first phone call.* When you decide to get help and you make the call for the appointment, you begin to think about what you will say. No doubt you imagine the therapist will ask what kind of help you're looking for or how they can best help you. Up until this point you may have had a lot of loose thoughts in your head about things that didn't feel right but that you hadn't crystallized, but now you need to respond with some sort of coherent description of the problem or challenge. Now you need to start thinking more concretely about what and why. Putting an issue into words, even inside your head, is the first step. Thus, just by deciding to make that first call, your therapy has begun. In fact, you, the reader, have already taken that step by buying this book. If you've read this far, I suspect you are further along, which leads me to say, "Welcome! Come on in! You're right on time for your appointment."

Chapter Three

Cooking Therapy: Effective and Efficient

Imagine this: It's the end of a rough day and you're tired or frustrated, unsure what to do with all those emotions bubbling up inside. Perhaps it's a Sunday and you're feeling anxious about the week ahead or, for that matter, anxious about anything. Take yourself into the kitchen and find a session recipe for calm, create one with calming ingredients of your own choosing, or pull out ingredients that you have on hand, without a trip to the store, and have an instant opportunity to relieve stress, anger, frustration, or sadness.

In this chapter we'll explore some of the many ways that cooking therapy is the perfect therapy for anyone, anytime—especially in the chaos of today's world. In addition to what you already know about the convenience of an experiential therapy that can be done at home, we'll look at how you can schedule it at a time that works for you and/or your family, for just the cost of the ingredients, and end up with a tangible and delicious representation of your session. We'll also look at how cooking therapy is great for every age. Then we'll take a closer look at how cooking therapy is great for folks looking to explore their relationships of any kind. And finally, we'll investigate how in this age of disconnect, cooking therapy can foster connection.

Cooking therapy does double duty. In other words, in addition to a new outlook, you'll have a snack or a meal. If you're going to prepare a dish or meal, it's easy to turn an ordinary cooking session into a healing event simply by pulling out the metaphors, being mindful, and applauding your mastery.

And while the food gives back calories and sustenance, it becomes clear that preparing our food gives back so much more; it gives us appreciation for our bodies and souls and immeasurable insight into ourselves. Cooking *therapy* gives us so much more. In each session, you'll be focused and mindful, you'll mine the steps for the metaphors that mirror your thoughts, behaviors, and feelings, and you'll contemplate what works and what doesn't. Just as a chef tastes a dish to see if it needs more or less of something, you will do the same for your relationships, sense of peace and balance, thoughts, feelings, and behaviors. In return, you'll not only have a dish you've mastered, but you'll have a mastery over your sense of self.

Cooking therapy is always there for you. Let's explore how this transformational therapy is ideal for all of us in this era of busy lives.

Making It Work for Your Timing

For many of us, life is busy, and we often have the sense that we're rushing around. It's hard to find the time to be still with ourselves for just a few moments and often even harder to schedule one more appointment, even if it might benefit our emotional well-being. The great news is that there are so many situations in life that can be improved by a cooking therapy session and so many ways to fit a session into your life.

For instance, some of us have a harried schedule in the morning and the thought of a therapy session seems impossible, but cooking therapy can be applied to a bowl of cereal as you notice the noise of the package, the softening of the flakes, the coolness of the milk—all done as you prepare and eat, with no extra time added. The same can be applied to a packaged yogurt or bar, which will have equally impactful metaphors. In other words, cooking therapy can even be done on the go! But let's look at some other scenarios that you may not have considered.

Ultimately, all of us have to eat something, and even if we're just reheating leftovers, a cooking therapy session is the perfect fit. In fact, *reheating* is a metaphor you may see often, especially if a relationship or situation has become stagnant. So, if you find that you have a little more time at lunch or the end of the day but you're tired and don't want to spend *too* much time, a cooking therapy session can be the perfect recipe for evaluating your day and even setting the tone for the next while also giving you your meal. Make that sandwich and you will explore layers in your relationships; toss a stir-fry and explore who or what you want to add or remove from your life; or warm up that leftover casserole and explore any old habits that are becoming too hardened. Other times, we may have time and energy on our hands. Perhaps your partner has a hobby or interest that you don't share, which leaves you with hours to fill. Or perhaps it's a weekend day and you're just bored and looking for a new way to self-explore. In these cases, a longer cooking therapy session can be the perfect fit. When we have the time to marinate, simmer, or chill, we have the opportunity to deeply explore the ways that those processes mirror our communication styles, our behavioral patterns, and our emotional reactions. In other words, no matter who you are or what your time constraints may be, cooking therapy will become your therapy concierge, available to you whenever you request it.

Cooking therapy also works from both the inside out (emotion) and outside in (setting or ingredients). In this book, you can choose the recipes provided based on topic or time. For example, if you have only a few minutes and are feeling low on self-esteem, you might choose the Fast Lane recipe in Chapter 7, "Infusing Confidence." If you are a bit stressed but have a leisurely day to cook, you might go for Scenic Drive in Chapter 6, "Creating Calm."

In addition to time, the subject matter of a session can be your guide. For example, if you've had a stressful day at work or even a confrontation with a colleague, you might choose a recipe that employs processes like chopping or pounding. Or you might have identified that you need to "bring down the heat" you're feeling and choose a recipe from Chapter 6, "Creating Calm." In that case you'll have recipes to choose from that are widely varied. Whenever a confrontation occurs, whether at work or home, in addition to feeling "heated internally," you may feel self-doubt or frustration that the episode did not go as planned. If this is the case, you may want to explore a short communication boost in Chapter 11, "How to Hear and Be Heard," or a new mindset in Chapter 8, "Radical Self-Acceptance."

All of us also have moments of sadness or malaise. They can arise from identifiable causes, like a breakup or a job loss, or be more amorphous, like a feeling of hopelessness or boredom. The next time you're feeling down, don't wallow or simply try to distract yourself. Get into the kitchen for a cooking therapy session of any length from Chapter 9, "Surviving Sadness." At times, we all need to sit with negative feelings, but let's also excavate them, decipher them, and put them back inside in a new way that has clarity and hope. We can't always remove sadness, but we can improve it. And don't forget, no need to commit to a multistep recipe or major culinary event, as you will find choices that take less than an hour or even just a few minutes, whatever works for you.

A common event that brings people into therapy is a looming change. It may be related to work or a new relationship or even parenthood. It may be another life stage such as a graduation, or perhaps a physical move to a different locale. But the universal emotions presented are doubt or fear. If you find yourself in this situation, cooking therapy is here for you. It's always helpful to try to tease out why you're trepidatious, and the tangible and concrete processes in a cooking therapy session are tailored to do just that. In the sessions in Chapter 7, "Infusing Confidence," and Chapter 10, "The Courage to Change," you will be infused with mastery and learn to melt away doubt. Rather than just talking about your ability to accomplish, you will have a visual representation of achievement. Through recipes chosen specifically to help you evaluate and consider your next moves, you'll create a new way of dealing with any changes that present themselves in the future.

In addition, if you are making a recipe of your own choosing, you can access Chapter 13, "Create Your Own Cooking Therapy Session," to see how to incorporate the 3M curriculum and therapeutic steps by using the ingredients of your choice or ones you have on hand. In other words, create your own cooking therapy session from your own recipe. Eventually, you'll be able to do this with ease, turning any recipe you choose into a customized cooking therapy session that "serves you well" and "fills you up."

All of the emotions and mental health challenges mentioned here, as well as others, will be further discussed in Chapter 4.

Perfect for All Ages

We talk often about the double-duty bonus in cooking therapy, but here's a little secret: There is a third benefit, and it's that cooking therapy is perfect for all ages, from very young children to senior citizens.

I've worked with children as young as four years old. One youngster comes to mind. Diego was four and a half, and his behaviors were out of control. His dad was responsible for discipline and rules, but he worked very long hours on varying shifts and was often gone on weekends. Diego was large for his age, and he would hit his seven-months-pregnant mother in the belly whenever he was frustrated or she said no to him. Consequently, she rarely set limits out of safety for the baby and herself, and Diego spent many hours in front of the television. Diego was also in danger. Because he didn't listen or have many rules, he would run out of the house into a fairly busy street. He would tease his mother that he was going to turn the knobs on their gas stove. It was truly a crisis situation, and I was a liaison with the family, the state-authorized provider, and the local division of youth and family services.

My sessions with Diego were illuminating. He liked when I came, and I realized quickly that he craved the attention. He also led me to a plastic playhouse in the family room, and we would sit in there and talk. I felt it was a bit of a physical metaphor for trying to contain himself, which bode well. He was content to spend an hour with me and had a great attention span for primitive questioning and book reading. But the minute we emerged, he would revert to being a wild child, running all over the house, not listening to his mother, throwing his food or snacks to the ground. Because of this, I felt that my sessions with Diego were merely using up time. If his mom couldn't make a change, neither would the situation. So I suggested a cooking therapy session. Most meals were prepared at home by his mom, but she'd never thought to include Diego. In fact, cooking and watching him was an ongoing challenge.

I think Diego's mother was skeptical, but Diego was excited when I showed up the next week with the ingredients for a microwave egg sandwich. I wanted something quick that would provide instant gratification but also show his mom that we could incorporate some positive participation, limit setting, and reward, choice, and applause. I certainly wasn't going to bring any sugar or energy bars into this intervention! Diego's mother had the eggs, sausage, cheese, and salsa. I brought ramekins, mini bagels, cooking spray, and baby spinach.

Diego loved placing the eggs and sausage in each ramekin. I modeled praise, and his mom followed suit. He was able to wait patiently for the eggs to be done (twenty seconds) and then helped sprinkle cheese. Each time, both his mom and I would provide lots of applause. Finally, we inverted it all onto a bagel with spinach, which Diego pulled off. We allowed him to do so but had him do it neatly. It was a positive experience.

While Diego's situation was complicated and might have required additional interventions and perhaps medication going forward, he was simply too young to diagnose or label, and at least his mother now had one tool she could embrace. When I saw Diego after that, he always wanted to cook, but even more, his mom had more awareness and guidance around reward language and limit setting. She reported that she was able to incorporate this type of cooking therapy into the family's day, that Diego even helped with some of the table setting, and that some of his outbursts had lessened, but she was also very much looking forward to all-day kindergarten!

Preteens and teens make some of the best cooking therapy participants, because they crave family activities more often than they let on. Additionally, both ages love an opportunity to exercise choice and be creative. In a family or supported cooking therapy session, clinical guidance should be as light and fluffy as a croissant and the focus on fun as heavy as a filled empanada. In other words, employing the 3M curriculum in a customized way will reap rewards.

Here are some examples: In attempting mindfulness, teens may be reluctant to "stop and look at the bowl of berries" for a full minute. Instead, you might ask them to notice the colors and guess whether the taste will be sweet or sour. Then you might prompt, "Name something in your day that's sweet and something that isn't." Don't dwell, unless they choose to, and move on. While teens may not want to focus on staring at anything for too long, they will smell and listen. With baking bread or chicken, smell can be used for further prompts. Questions such as "What memories does this bring up?" can lead to a discussion of lost feelings and the desire to reclaim or add them. Frying or sizzling can provoke similar conversation. If parents are fully participating, they should add their thoughts. Finally, just the process of participation as well as the finished product are representative of mastery, and parents should affirm this; everyone should applaud the effort and result to inspire pride. Let each child or teen choose a name for the recipe used. Even a little happy dance for celebration will provoke smiles.

Children and teens are surprisingly good at cooking therapy when it is couched as a game. The more they "play" at it, the better they will become at teasing out the metaphors, noticing the mindful moments, and feeling accomplished. Remember, this is their and your activity. As long as a session doesn't mirror being forced to practice piano or watch their sister's soccer game, children and teens will become fully engaged and grow in terms of mindful behaviors and feelings.

Additionally, cooking therapy is an excellent opportunity for adults to process their feelings. Jenna is a married, forty-year-old mom of two children, ages ten and fourteen, who came to a group cooking therapy session sponsored by a book club. The topic for the session was chosen by the club moderator as "parenting issues." Many of the women were experiencing stress from perceived competition with other moms of similarly aged kids who were all in school together. Jenna offered that she sometimes felt she didn't measure up and was constantly comparing herself to others in terms of her kids' accomplishments at school, their after-school activities, and their college readiness pursuits, and even in terms of her own clothes, car, and house. Many of the women were silent, but some concurred.

The group session was structured so that the women worked in pairs. Each time a task was performed, each member of the pair would have one minute to share something with the other. For example, when peeling a cucumber, the prompt might be for each person in the pair to reveal to the other a feeling or behavior they'd like to lose or felt they had lost, especially as it might relate to feelings of a lack of self-confidence or competence. Working with olives provided the metaphor of "a pit in your stomach," which acted as a prompt for further sharing feelings along those lines, but also offered the opportunity to recall a sense of accomplishment in terms of "pitting" a tough situation.

Once the cooking therapy discussion was over, an additional processing session took place. Many of the women, including Jenna, expressed that they had no idea other women felt exactly the same way and had similar doubts and fears, and they even shared ideas for feeling better about themselves and letting go of negative self-doubt. All took something positive from the session and especially loved the mastery inherent in having a physical representation of their wellness work.

At a women's wellness and empowerment retreat, a group session addressing the challenge of life transitions was offered to women who were empty nesting and entering a new life stage. While some were excited to seek new opportunities, spend time with a partner, or explore a hobby, all were wondering about filling endless hours and changing roles. Alice, one of the older participants, had had her children later in life than most and expressed that she felt too old to start anything new but was afraid of being unnecessary or useless. Using a recipe that involved stuffing and unstuffing, I was able to lead the women through the idea of becoming comfortable with change.

First, mini cucumbers were halved and scooped out to suggest "empty" nesting and to make "boats" that would be fresh and ready to receive new ideas and endeavors. The cucumber was saved on the side. In a cooking therapy session, when you scoop out, it should always remind you that an empty vessel is abundantly ready to be filled with something new. With no kitchen available, the recipe I chose called for a filling that would simulate a bagel with lox and cream cheese while inspiring chances and choices. Spreading cream cheese gave the participants a chance to think about what they might like to "spread" into their lives and also set the base for accepting new ideas that would stick. Alice offered that while she didn't "expect to be taking up painting or anything else like that," she did love to read and might have more time for some of the books piled up on her nightstand. Other women talked about how they might travel, volunteer, or learn a language. Small pieces of smoked salmon were minced and placed on the cream cheese to acknowledge that feeling a little like you are in bits and pieces after a life change is perfectly normal. The women were asked to sit for a mindful minute with that acceptance. In order to move forward, I explained, it's important to acknowledge how you feel with as much clarity and specificity as possible. Many offered that being able to say out loud that they did feel less "whole" was the most powerful part of the session. Next, I used tomatoes to represent evolution, as the gelatinous insides suggested that they were still in a developmental stage. All were asked to chop the tomatoes and think about embracing the idea of developing and evolving and filling themselves with that concept rather than focusing on what was scooped out. But then I asked the women to chop bits of the reserved cucumber and sprinkle them onto the tomatoes to represent that everyone's children were still present in their lives and not lost. We also took a mindful moment to acknowledge the cucumber seeds, which could represent seeds of change. Alice said she'd never thought of change as anything but upsetting. I asked her to focus on the brightness of the cucumber flesh and to try to change her vision of change as dark and disturbing and flip a switch in her mind to imagine change as bright and green. She agreed to try.

Finally, we sprinkled everything-bagel seasoning on the boats, and the metaphor was clear: Everything can be ahead of you, and the future may even be spicy and delicious! The women were all encouraged to "take a bite" out of considering their new roles and to keep their new boats afloat. I named this session "Smooth Sailing Cucumber Boats." Alice came over to me privately after the session and said that she was surprised at how cooking therapy had lessoned her uncertainty and anxiety and made her feel more comfortable than she'd expected.

Cooking Therapy for Relationships of All Kinds

It would be wonderful if every relationship could be brought into the kitchen and explored through a cooking therapy session. The results would be exponentially successful in creating communication and relationship wellness. If possible, you should bring your siblings or your parents or even your in-laws, if you dare, into a session. Issues with friends? The kitchen can be your canvas to open up honest communication. All of the clinical benefits of cooking therapy, such as working side by side, sharing tasks, disconnecting from distractions, and the 3M principles, can be effective at teasing out feelings and promoting communication.

However, even if you can't get a partner or friend to participate, these relationships can benefit from a cooking therapy session; you will just have to tackle the relationship and communication issues by yourself. But that's not bad news. Replaying an issue with a colleague through the cooking therapy lens can be quite helpful. Once you get comfortable and seasoned as your own sous therapist™, you might even try a technique we discussed earlier from gestalt and perform the whole cooking therapy session as if you are the other person. But that's for later. For now, just know that with this book, you'll learn to tackle any relationship and communication issues on your own.

A Soothing Balm for the Epidemic of Disconnect in the Modern Era

A wonderful benefit of cooking therapy has been the unexpected joy that young and old clients feel from an activity that does not involve bells, buzzers, beeps, ringtones, or other sounds associated with technology. Cooking therapy is much like a walk in the woods, where you might sit by a stream, notice the trees, feel the breeze, listen to the waves, smell the salt air. Every single one of our natural senses can be activated in cooking therapy. We notice the pour of the milk, feel the heat from the oven, listen to the water boiling, and smell the baking bread. Nothing could be more connective to nature than nourishing and nurturing our minds through our bodies. Even Buddha said, "When we prepare our own food, we give to the food and the food gives back."

This wisdom played out in a virtual cooking therapy session with a writer for *Bon Appétit* magazine. We both agreed that technology addiction was on the rise, and she was looking for new and different ways to quell her own anxiety and suspected that cell phones and tablets and days of laptop sitting were partially to blame. We shared our kitchens through our screens as I took her through the steps, and typical of any therapy session, there were moments of discomfort. Excavating feelings and habits can be painful at first. During the session, she reported that her discomfort soon turned to revelations through, of all things, zoodles, and as she separated them she came to some surprising conclusions about her connections, especially to food. New perspectives on herself were revealed to her, as well as moments of mindfulness and mastery. Going forward, she shared that her takeaway was that an activity you can do several times a day, every day, that can help you look at life in an honest way, has to be helpful. She left the session with new ideas and feelings about herself, and I left trusting that she would be able to handle the effects of technology use and that the new skills she'd learned would aid in conquering fears and act as an antidote to anxiety in all areas.

It's no secret that psychologists across the world are warning about the effects of too much technology on mood and mind. Our children and teens are struggling with eye contact and social cues and relying too much on social media to determine how they feel about themselves. Therapists are seeing anxiety in record numbers and in increasingly young children. One psychiatric school in New Jersey, Cornerstone Day School, has a record number of psychiatrically fragile kids and a robust school phobia program. The school reports that guidance counselors from all over the state have been encouraging the administration to open additional resources for children as young as kindergarten. Some of this is due to the disconnect from COVID, but it had begun years before and can be attributed to the rewiring of our kids to text more and play less.

Psychologist Jonathan Haidt calls this "the great rewiring of childhood" in his book *The Anxious Generation*. Haidt describes how "play-based childhood" began to decline in the 1980s and how it was finally wiped out by the arrival of "phone-based childhood" in the early 2010s. He presents more than a dozen mechanisms by which this "great rewiring of childhood" has interfered with children's social and neurological development, covering everything from sleep deprivation to attention fragmentation, addiction, loneliness, social contagion, social comparison, and perfectionism.

Thanks to the internet and cell phones, we can always be reached. Much has been studied about the effects of this on both children and adults. The effects of social media have led therapists to begin diagnosing on-call syndrome (OCS) in both children and adults.

For children and teens, constant checking of social media sites creates FOMO (fear of missing out) and presents an unrealistic view of their peers, who may seem happier, prettier, more popular, and to be having more fun. And yet, despite this, teens also experience FOBO (fear of being offline). It's a lose-lose. They are both afraid to be missing out and need to know if they are. This can lead to obsessive doomscrolling and countless hours online.

Constant social media exposure is directly related to negative self-image and self-esteem, anxiety, depression, and suicide in teens. According to the *Journal of the American Academy of Psychiatry and Law*, researchers uncovered that the incidences of both cyberbullying and adolescent suicide are rising in the United States, with recent Centers for Disease Control and Prevention data showing that 14.9 percent of adolescents have been cyberbullied and 13.6 percent of adolescents have made a serious suicide attempt (Schonfeld, 2023).

Former US surgeon general Dr. Vivek Murthy described the rising suicide rates as a national emergency and called for a warning label on social media sites like those on cigarettes. "The more time an adolescent spends online, the greater the impact on their mental health," said Murthy. "Adolescents who spend more than three hours a day on social media face double the <u>risk</u> of anxiety and depression symptoms, and the average daily use in this age group was 4.8 hours, as of the summer of 2023. Additionally, nearly half of adolescents in this age group say social media makes them feel worse about their bodies" (Shah, 2024).

For adults, OCS takes on a different shape. We grown-ups can always be reached by a family member or a robotic call but especially by a boss, and we never have the chance to truly unwind and recharge. A study in *Scientific American* links extended work availability with decreased calmness, mood, and energy levels (Turner, 2016). If we are unavailable, it may be seen as undedicated or lazy. If a colleague is more available, perhaps they will receive an opportunity or promotion. And yet, one hour of disconnect does not cause the world to fall apart. Rather, it has the opposite effect. Adults relish the chance to reality-check their fears and anxieties, and after one cooking therapy session they are often recharged, balanced, and empowered to perform even more effectively.

Another syndrome being recognized by psychologists is PAS, or partially aware syndrome. There is new data to suggest that because we can be reached and reach out all the time, we're never fully involved in any activity. Often, the temptation to check our phone is just too compelling. With so many pings, pongs, beeps, bells, and ringtones associated with technology, we have to know if there's a message waiting for us.

Imagine a new mother who is nursing hears someone else's baby cry. Not only might she think it's her child, but the association is so powerful that if she is breastfeeding, her "letdown" response kicks in and she's ready to nurse. This is now being replicated with cell phones; the power of gadget sounds is causing many of us to continually check and check in with our own phones. It's like a technological letdown response.

In terms of being present, connected, and engaged, we're all aware of the example of a family in a restaurant where no one is talking to each other because even children as young as two are on iPads or cell phones. Without checks and balances, Ms. Rachel and *Peppa Pig* can quickly become more compelling than Mom and Dad. Think about the long-term effects this lack of verbal and nonverbal interactions, eye contact, and facial cues may have on child development.

Teens are especially reluctant to give up their phones. One sixteen-year-old client told me he'd rather be suspended and grounded than give up his cell phone. Instead of in-person experiences, his world was ruled by social media and an online sphere of influence. Instead of sleeping, he was scrolling way after his parents thought he was asleep. His parents were contacted and told that he'd been falling asleep in class. They had no idea that their son was so addicted and, going forward, set limits on his use.

The good news is that every time I've had a child or teen in a cooking therapy session, they've flourished. If there is any initial hesitation, it gives way to comfort and joy, and you can see them forget about their phones and notice a relief at not being "on call" for the next ping. If you are a parent or have children in your life in any way, or if these attributes remind you of anyone you love, including yourself, you can incorporate cooking therapy into your life every day to counteract the tension of tech.

Activities where children or adults can put down their phones and engage with family, community, and self-expression is the answer. We only have to implement the change. Experiential experiences are not only needed more than ever, but they are essential for bringing connection back to families and increasing health and wellness. Cooking therapy does just that.

Psychologists and clinicians report that clients who engage in a digital detox show signs of increased self-awareness and attention span as well as a reduction in stress and anxiety. The skills you learn in this book will allow you to address that disconnect and improve your mental health naturally as you go about your day by taking advantage of the many opportunities to perform a cooking therapy session through your regular preparations of meals and snacks.

By putting down your phone and picking up your ladle or spatula, you'll be more present, more mindful, and more self-confident and infuse yourself with pride in your own accomplishments, rather than comparing yourself to the memes and posts online and ending up with damaging self-perceptions. In the next chapter, we'll address many of the negative and pervasive emotions so many of us face, and I'll explain to you how cooking therapy can address them all.

Chapter Four

A "Recipe" for Almost Everything

In the chapters ahead we'll explore ways to create calm, banish self-doubt, increase self-esteem, add positivity to your life, explore change, and improve communication. With the triple components of mindfulness, metaphors, and mastery, you'll be able to address all of these areas every single day. When it comes to creating calm and balance in your life, there are purposeful cooking therapy processes that instantly address those internal feelings of rushing or swirling as well as emotions like fear, dread, or panic that can be incapacitating. In terms of self-confidence and self-doubt, you will leave every cooking therapy session with a newfound strength of spirit and self-worth, just by completing the session, which can be as short as five to ten minutes. Working with metaphors is an unbelievably powerful clinical process that will fulfill you in the session and stick with you once the session is over, not just for the day but as you go through most situations in the future. Imagine addressing these underlying self-doubts and seeing them morph into confidence and clarity and the strength it takes to evaluate or make a change. These are just some of the benefits of cooking therapy that you'll integrate.

But first, let's talk a little about some of the other emotional challenges that cooking therapy can specifically help.

Sadness

If you have been dealing with sadness due to life transitions, boredom, or a sense that something needs to change, cooking therapy is the perfect tool to dig into what's beneath the surface.

When sadness is the motivating reason to seek help, it's important to know that you're not alone. The rates of sadness and depression rose sharply during the pandemic, and isolation has been shown to be a key contributor, along with job loss, financial insecurity, and life events. The National Institutes of Health report a sharp increase in depression and a continued rise in rates each year.

Cooking therapy can help to target and alleviate the overall feelings of sadness you may be experiencing as well as some specific causes. A common thread with sorrow, especially sorrow that is of new onset but pervasive, is a longing for former homeostasis, the ability to function and feel "normal," and the associated loss of self-worth as a client imagines themselves, wrongly, to be defective. If that is what you're feeling right now, you will find solace in the sessions designed specifically for surviving sadness.

Sometimes sadness is due to mourning and grief. In dealing with loss of life, the client mourns their loved one as well as their vision or plan for how the future would unfold. In cooking therapy, we don't minimize the weight of the feeling, no matter the cause. You'll be able to identify your experience of sadness, normalize your individual reactions, and even develop a timeline for moving forward. With cooking therapy, you have a built-in support group and a comfort zone.

When working with a client where sadness is due to loss, I often use "disappearing" ingredients that inform the recipe even though the taste is no longer present. For instance, there are cookie recipes that use a teaspoon of molasses, not a very tasty ingredient on its own. It's hugely important for consistency, but the taste "goes away." This is a great metaphor for confronting loss without losing the pleasure once associated with that person or situation before the loss. In this way, it's not just the loss that's overwhelming every emotion; there is balance. Similarly, we often use salt in baking to enhance flavor and strengthen the dough. Though you won't taste the salt, it's still very present, informing the total dish, and that's a great metaphor for keeping a lost loved one's spirit alive.

Another example would be a "reduction." Think about balsamic vinegar being the base of a sauce that is "burned off"; while no longer present, it deepens the taste and richness of the dish. That's a strong metaphor for positive memory. In other words, a person or version of a person who is no longer here can still be seen as enriching even though only a "hint" remains. The message is that only a hint, while so sad, is not without worth.

Sometimes sadness is due to situations that can't change but that can be reframed. When this is the case, I've been known to script a "failure" into a session to highlight a change in perspective. The end result of the session may be a fallen cake, a burnt caramel sauce, or an overcooked chicken. Each of these items may initially seem like a disaster that can't be salvaged, but that's the beauty of cooking therapy; not only is there mastery in a dish that comes out perfectly, but there is mastery in learning to see the journey as the important part and the end result as what you make of it. The cake can be turned into a delicious pudding, the caramel into candy bars, and the chicken diced for chicken salad or tacos. Sometimes you have to sit with your situation. But that doesn't mean you have to sit with never-ending sadness. Reframe. Repurpose. Relax.

Years ago, I worked with a family that had two children. One child was constantly in trouble and had been diagnosed with attention deficit/hyperactivity disorder (ADHD). The parents were so stuck for so long asking themselves why their child who misbehaved more often "wasn't like their other child." They were grieving the "loss" of two "perfect" daughters, which was hurting everyone. Slowly, we began to explore whether the loss was actually a complete one and whether or not there were any "wins."

Eventually I was able to help them see that the "challenging" child contributed to them in ways they didn't realize. For instance, they grew compassionate and non-judgmental of other parents and children and more relatable to these same folks. They developed the creativity necessary to address their other child's needs and grew in ways they hadn't realized.

In this way, change, or the need to adjust one's perspective or lifestyle, can mirror loss.

Along this line, another cooking therapy recipe might be the addition of an ingredient that is distasteful on its own, such as the molasses or salt, but does give a dish "layers." Other examples might be cinnamon or Worcestershire sauce. When working through these issues, I would likely choose a recipe with ingredients like these, which are somewhat awful alone but, with time and heat, do contribute, and the bitterness either is absorbed or even flavors the dish. It's a powerful example of "different" being contributory.

All of these causes for sadness can be addressed with cooking therapy. In Chapter 9, "Surviving Sadness," you will have the chance to address your situation and improve your mood. You'll be amazed at the way a tangible activity can crystallize or uncover the root of your emotion.

Anxiety and Stress

Just as sadness and depression have increased over time, so has stress and anxiety, and this rise is manifesting in young children and teens as well as adults.

While many of us have felt stress in varying degrees at work and home and in family relationships through the years, there are newer causes, much of them externally caused, that are the culprits. In the last twenty years, terrorism and war have been on the rise, as are random acts of violence in previously safe spaces, such as schools, movie theaters, shopping malls, and restaurants. The use of benzodiazepines, the so-called "calming drugs" like Valium and Xanax, has risen sharply in the last two decades.

You are not alone if you're feeling like you or your loved ones are experiencing a lot of anxiety and stress, or if you're experiencing generalized anxiety disorder, panic attacks, or panic disorder.

In cooking therapy, we address anxiety and stress, including the internally driven causes of stress that may be due to negative self-talk, self-critique, or low self-esteem, in a complete and wraparound way. First, we take a look at the level of anxiety you feel by recognizing it. In a cooking therapy session, there is no need to hide or pretend that you're not anxious; in fact, we will sit with it mindfully, choose recipes to address it specifically, and ultimately cook through it by using the ingredients and processes that target uncomfortable feelings and convert them to calm, peace, and balance. When it comes to negative self-talk, we excavate the learned falsehood through peeling or scooping and generalize it to self-talk going forward.

While externally driven stressors are often out of our control, internally driven stress may be due to a variety of reasons. Sometimes it's simply a response to those external events, while at other times these fears or anxieties are implanted in childhood. Still other causes are genetic. With cooking therapy, we can tease out the commonalities in all of these instances and address the feelings. For example, some clients may worry that they won't be able to successfully complete the session. We reality-check that fear by working together to accomplish our cooking goals and use that mastery to reality-check some other erroneous fears, like a terror attack in the neighborhood.

Some fears are in a class of their own. Fears and phobias are considered one of the easier mental health issues to treat through a process called desensitization. For example, fear of flying may be approached by first looking at planes in a magazine, then in a video, then at a private airport, and eventually by boarding a plane and ultimately taking an actual flight. Couple this with relaxation and breathing techniques, and the chance for success is high. The same methods might apply to fear of spiders, heights, or crowded spaces. As the client becomes more anxious, the therapist infuses calming techniques and reality testing into the process so the client can move forward.

In cooking therapy, we can address anxiety, false thinking, and helplessness by teasing out the fears with metaphors and creating mindful moments. For instance, there are recipes, such as pudding or candy, where waiting or patiently stirring is necessary until a consistency or temperature is reached. This can model "sitting with the feeling or fear." Even waiting for a pot of water to boil can mirror the "bubbling up" of anxiety. It can then be lessened by simply lowering the heat—or deescalating the situation. These can be used to model the vulnerability or sense of being out of control and return that power to the client. If you experience fears or phobias, recipes that require a dish to rest, marinate, or thicken require a waiting period, which mirrors the moments in desensitization where you may wait and breathe through moments.

Chapters 6, 7, and 8 of *Cooking as Therapy* will help guide you toward inner calm, infused confidence, and a road map for loving yourself just the way you are as you work through anxiety and stress.

The Holidays

Peace and joy on earth, right? Sure, sometimes. But not every family is so lucky during the holidays. Some of the stories I've heard go like this:

- "My brother and sister had a big fight, and she stormed out."
- "The minute my mom walked in, she told me I looked fat."

- "My son's new girlfriend was dressed for the beach."
- "I was so worried something would go wrong, I forgot to turn on the oven."

So many scenarios can cause stress at the holidays. Often, it begins weeks in advance. We may be worried about unexpected mishaps or feel pressure to create that perfect Norman Rockwell experience: white tablecloth with no stains, well-behaved and drama-free relatives, perfectly browned and juicy turkey or golden apple pie. Sounds more like a fabricated beer commercial than real life, and it applies to even nontraditional holidays like Mother's Day or Halloween. Don't even get me started on being single on Valentine's Day! It takes a real tough cookie to handle the stress.

Before major holidays, try fortifying yourself in advance with Zen-like dishes such as rice pudding. You could name it "The Aloof Is in the Pudding," or "Who's Been Naughty or Rice Pudding." Puddings necessitate patience and stirring and require you to stir gently, which will remind you not to "stir things up." Eventually, puddings need to chill. The pudding comes together in the fridge, and it's an excellent visual for "coming together" at any holiday or other potentially stressful family event. Even a chilled pudding may seem a little wobbly, and that's a metaphor too. You don't counteract a lifetime of family dynamics in one day or one dish. Still, wobbly or shaky, it holds, and you will too.

One word about bringing up hot topics at holiday meals: Don't! It doesn't matter who you're voting for, what religion you're newly following, or how much money you made this year. And no one really cares that the neighbor's child identifies as a cat. Toward that end, I have a handy cooking therapy metaphor system. I encourage you to consider the Scoville scale for measuring the amount of heat in peppers before you bring up a "hot topic." Think about the various peppers you know and how some are superhot (avoid), while others are hot but tolerable (proceed cautiously) and some peppers are not hot at all (yes, please!). With the Scoville technique, the hotter the pepper, the more sugar and water solution is needed to dilute it, and this is how the pepper is rated. If you apply the Scoville scale to the topics at your family dinners and continually add sweetness to the hottest subjects, I promise you, there will be fewer jalapeños and many more bells.

Anger, Resentment, and Frustration

Cooking therapy is especially effective when it comes to processing anger. Anger isn't always a negative emotion. In fact, it can be more damaging *not* to express healthy anger. The difference between healthy and unhealthy anger often has to do with reflection. If you can respond without being emotionally reactive or process feelings thoughtfully and still feel angry, not only is your point of view more likely to be heard, but your anger will exhale rather than become trapped inside your body and mind, creating emotional and physical symptoms.

Anger, resentment, and frustration can become pathological, meaning they are no longer situational and fleeting but rather permanent, destructive, and debilitating. If these emotions have moved in and taken root in your emotional nest, it's time for action.

In my experience, resentment is usually not a momentary reaction; rather, it builds and is more layered, often the result of anger or frustration about a situation. Here are some examples: A colleague at work is promoted to a position you thought you deserved. You may feel anger or hurt first, which grows into feelings of resentment. Or maybe your in-laws are constantly showering your newly married daughter with pricey gifts you can't afford to give. You may want to feel happy for her, and you do, but you also feel multiple other emotions that may include anger, sadness, envy, and perhaps even misplaced shame. In an effort to manage all of these feelings, resentment builds. And it's not because her in-laws are bad people; it's because it's all happening inside you and because of how you're processing it. This could determine your relationship with your daughter and her new family in the future, so what you choose to feel and how you act upon those feelings are important. The same is true for the work colleague that got promoted. They didn't do anything wrong, and perhaps your resentment is toward the supervisor, but if you don't process your feelings in a way that makes them palatable, the impact could be even worse than losing the promotion: If you go forward feeling resentful, it can poison your performance, self-worth, and happiness at work.

The good news is that there are cooking therapy processes and sessions to address all of these feelings. You might create a "reduction" or learn to "bring down the heat." You may be smashing small potatoes or pounding chicken breasts. You may also be sifting through flour or beans and gaining clarity on what you feel and why you feel the way you do. And blending sugar and butter, or different spices for a rub, will guide you toward the understanding that two emotions can occupy the same space and be tolerable. So you can feel happy that your daughter has generous in-laws and admit to a bit of envy but lose the resentment as you add in the benefits, such as her happiness and secure future and the fact that her in-laws adore her—and you may solidify this in session with add-ins like vanilla, chocolate chips, or cinnamon. Add-ins are a great metaphor, and you'll use them often to soften negativity. These and many other techniques will be your armor and your sword against anger and resentment. The concrete tasks and visual results will guide you toward understanding your thoughts and feelings and promote healthier habits and behaviors.

When it comes to frustration, levels are on the rise. An article in *Psychology Today* cites a 2023 Gallup emotions poll that found frustration and other negative emotions to be at the highest levels ever counted. We tend to think of frustration as a feeling that percolates just below the surface. Although frustration may cause lashing out, it's often less reactive, like resentment, and tolerated for longer, which is both the good and bad news. All of us need to temper our emotions in response to minor and fleeting events. When we learn to let these small annoyances burn off the way we might let alcohol in a sauce burn off, we remain calm, and this serves us well emotionally. On the other hand, if both small and large frustrations are "baked" into our daily bread, it will be awfully hard for us to be peaceful or joyful.

In cooking therapy, frustration is tackled through the use of processes and steps with no pressure for perfection and increased tolerance of imperfections. Mindfulness is implemented in every recipe, which is a powerful antidote to the seething or bubbling you may feel below the surface. Additionally, you will incorporate impactful metaphors and physically peel away layers as you peel away the hard and cemented feelings that are keeping you from letting go. And these cooking therapy sessions will stay with you long after the session ends to remind you of a lighter you.

Additionally, if anger, resentment, or frustration has become learned as an inner and constant feeling unattached to anything specific, has been integrated as a personality trait, or even functions as a go-to communication response, cooking therapy can help by rewiring self-talk to create new feelings, infusing calm into reactions and responses and presenting real and new choices for better and more positive actions and habits.

Sometimes other scenarios are responsible for entrenching anger and resentment in an individual or family. Common emotions include anger that one individual is taking up all the emotional, physical, or financial resources and resentment of the family member as well as others in the family who are accommodating. At the same time, there may be some shame in acknowledging that emotion, since the less needy individual is deemed to be the "lucky" one. Conversely, sometimes the individual is the sufferer, and they are managing anger and frustration of their own as well as large lumps of shame. In all of these scenarios, you will see how cooking therapy shines a new light on the picture and adds tools for dealing with current and future occurrences of rage and disappointment. Ingredients that require clarifying, reducing, or opening allow feelings to be spoken and shared. Processes such as chopping, pounding, and pureeing mirror healthy outlets for anger.

Cooking therapy will provide you with a road map for reflection and thoughtfulness. You will be instructed to perform each step purposefully, not blindly, with thought and deliberation, exploring old patterns and creating new ones as needed.

Examples of Cooking Therapy Recipes for Everyday Challenges

One of the most wonderful aspects of cooking therapy is that it can be used as an immediate salve or Band-Aid for a life event or situation. A cooking therapy session can inject humor and perspective into the most frustrating life events. Below are some examples of everyday frustrations. Some or all may resonate with you. As you have learned, it's important to name your recipes for "stickiness" once the session is over. I've given you examples of how to do that in each of these "pretend" sessions. As you read the short hypothetical situations, practice naming each with a recipe of your own choosing. This will begin to prepare you for doing the same when you're conducting a cooking therapy session in your own home.

1. **Feeling stressed that you can't do it all or are juggling too many roles?** There's a recipe for that! Hint: It's something super easy to make that looks fabulous, like "Dishwasher Salmon." Yes, you heard me right: You make it in the dishwasher, and yes, you will choose the "quick wash" cycle. For the busy cook, it's a simple dish that takes almost no work,

pioneered by Bob Blumer, host of Food Network's *The Surreal Gourmet*. But the powerful metaphor is how simplifying some aspects of your life can actually create a better dish. So, pop on some dill and a two ingredient crème fraîche, wrap the salmon in foil, and let the self-applause fill you with a new resolve to feed your soul as well as your many roles. And of course, we'll rename this recipe "Simply Superb Simplified Salmon."

2. **Is a colleague stealing your thunder?** Or do you have a boss that makes you feel inadequate? Advocating for yourself at work is tricky. These situations happen all the time, and there are many manuals on office politics to guide you toward empowerment. But I vote for "Give Me Credit Crème Brûlée." In this recipe you start with "small" dishes (ideas) and a cool base, much as you would when you begin a conversation or suggest a change at work. Be confident but cool and calm. Becoming too emotional at work or in any discussion rarely serves you well, and hot crème brûlée wouldn't either. But then seal the dish and your resolve by caramelizing the top. There's nothing like a blowtorch to get your confidence up and your sense of power back.

3. I recall one session with a woman whose **husband was constantly belittling her**, with a little bit of gaslighting thrown in, too. Do you remember the group session for divorced women where we chopped sausages? I hope you're laughing at that one; it's a reminder that humor has its place even in serious work. We named that recipe "Cuts Less Deep Sausage and Onions."

4. **Truly divorcing?** When it comes to the ending of a relationship, modeling the universality of breakups leads me to suggest a recipe that's common and familiar. You can incorporate "separating" egg whites from their yolks, because that's the reality. An easy way to remove any pieces of cracked shell that sneak in is with a bit of water on your finger, which not only mirrors removing the "sharp shells" of the relationship but also demonstrates how "diluting" isn't ruining the dish but helping. Additionally, you can channel a "reduction," which is so intensely flavorful, like "Strong and Single Sauce"—because "reducing" does not have to mean "less than," and with time can mean much more.

5. **New parent?** No doubt you're overwhelmed, not only because of the many emotional changes but also physically, from lack of sleep. I like to invent recipe names and then create a dish, and you can too. You'd probably want to make "I Need Coffee Cake," then find a coffee cake recipe. I also love the idea of shaping or "role-ing" meatballs into *cocktail* size (because you'll probably need one), and the size will represent the little one who is now a big presence in your life. You could name them "My Life Is 'Sweetish' Meatballs" and search for a recipe for cocktail or Swedish meatballs. New parents will also benefit from approaches that help with grief and loss, as this is a major life transition. There can be feelings of loss of self as well as loss of body. Just after I had my first child, I went to get a new pair of nonpregnancy jeans. I found a pair that fit (barely), but when I brought them home, I noticed the tag; it said Buffalo Brand, which made me cry, because my

body was still so large that I felt just like a buffalo! And when I worked at a women's wellness center, there was one new mom who shared that when she came home from the hospital, she cried every day in the shower, letting the water mix with her tears. I would have loved to make a pudding soufflé for both of us and watch the molten pudding slowly drip to mirror all the emotions spilling out, but we definitely wouldn't have had the time! An on-target recipe is a one-minute egg, where you can watch as the yolk spills out. Just name it "I Am Still Egg-celent!"

6. **Elderly or retiring?** You may be despondent at this life change and need a recipe that's empowering, a recipe that says life is different but not over and taps into your years of wisdom. How great would it be to make a crust out of Wise potato chips to reinforce your considerable knowledge and remind you not to get "old and crusty" or stale? Toward that end, I'd also attempt something challenging, like a recipe on the cover of *Bon Appétit* magazine. Why something so challenging? Because you're up to it! (And let's face it, you have the time.) This is one session where I'd also suggest making bread. It takes time, some expertise, and patience, all of which you likely have in stock. You might even name the recipe first— perhaps "Roll With It Rolls From Scratch"—and then find a bread or rolls recipe that intrigues you.

7. **Toxic friends?** If you have a large circle of friends, it can be tough to unload just one. You can try to be diplomatic, but often a friend who is passive-aggressive, critical, or outright sabotaging will not have the awareness to recognize and change their patterns. One of my clients reported that her good

friend was always saying things like "It's a good thing you have me to remember things for you, because your brain is like a sieve!" If you've tried to explain nicely that your feelings are hurt but with no result, it may be time for more drastic tactics. Good friends are supposed to make you feel good about yourself. If they are infectious or worrisome, I liken it to a lump or mass: Try the topical treatments, then the more invasive radiation and chemotherapy. But if nothing's working, it may be time for surgery to cut it out. Remember, when it comes to specific circumstances, we'll be able to pull out the common feelings of fear, malaise, frustration, sadness, and any other negative emotions that occur in situational issues or events and attack them. A recipe for toxic friends should give a nod to toxins—not real ones, please. A mélange of mushrooms, softened in a pan, will fit the bill. I suggest we call this recipe "You Can't Hurt Me Any *Spore*."

A Note about Eating Disorders

Eating disorders should never be treated with cooking therapy unless the client is well into their recovery and assisted by a licensed and trained eating disorders specialist. You may wonder why cooking therapy should not at least be used to spark calm and confidence, or the teased-out commonalities, in these cases as in other challenging circumstances we've discussed. Whatever the specific diagnosis, the associations with food are so intrinsic to the issues and the results not only emotionally but potentially medically dangerous that it's best to avoid any culinary therapy unless it is highly monitored and supervised and, once again, determined to be appropriate by a skilled eating disorders professional.

Are you ready to try cooking therapy? I hope you now feel prepared and excited, as I suspect that you will never cook the same way again after today. And that's a good thing. If we can try to make everything we do more conscious and purposeful and self-reflective, even the things we never thought of as therapeutic, like cooking, that's a recipe for emotional success.

As your Sous Therapist™, I've individualized each session to meet your culinary and emotional needs or preferences. For example, these sessions can use kosher, gluten-free, dairy-free, or vegan ingredients. They can also address most common mental health issues like anxiety, depression, relational problems, and the "common threads" of the many more complex disorders. Again, experiential therapies have been shown to augment traditional therapy rather than replace it. These recipes will also help with the "situational issues" I've delineated, such as office politics, empty nesting, marital differences, and ways to be heard, as well as many more too numerous to list.

From gathering the ingredients to noticing the result, we will explore the many actions in cooking that mirror our learned patterns in life. Do you struggle with patience or attention to detail? Are you averse to new things or striving for perfection? So many of our behaviors become apparent when we cook, if we're paying attention. Some serve us well, while others hold us back. Identifying the difference can be a breakthrough experience.

With *Cooking as Therapy*, you will have multiple opportunities to target or explore a behavior, pattern, or communication style. Whether you use the recipe sessions provided or one of your own choosing, the ingredients and cooking methods can all contribute to self-exploration and insight. Let's begin.

Chapter Five

How to Use This Book

In this chapter, I'll walk you through the process of cooking therapy, whether you are making your own recipe and would like to infuse a little cooking therapy into your dinner preparation or whether you would like a guided recipe that I've written. I'll explain how cooking therapy sessions work, outline the rules of any cooking therapy session, and walk you through some metaphors and tools for working with the most common cooking methods and ingredients that you can apply to your own cooking routine.

Chapters 6 through 11 each include one recipe in each of the three categories below, for a total of three recipes apiece, to target a topic based on the amount of time you choose to spend.

- **Fast Lane:** Recipes that require little or no cooking and take ten to fifteen minutes
- **Easy Rider:** Recipes that take up to one hour, including cooking time
- **Scenic Drive:** Recipes that may require chilling or marinating and are intended for a leisurely experience with an open-ended amount of time

The lessons learned in a cooking therapy session should not end once a dish is done. Together we need to "make enough" to have leftovers! In other words, I give you the tools to remember and implement the lessons learned long after the session is over. To give each session "glue" or "legs," I'll give you a to-go bag of all the essential points, so you'll have an easy way to reference the steps you took and the insights you've gained.

At the end of each section, you can savor an "After-Dinner Mint." This is just a reminder that all lessons have an impact at different times. Though some revelations occur during session, others need to marinate before the flavor appears. This is true for any therapy session, be it traditional or experiential. It may be hours, days, or weeks later that an *aha* or lightbulb moment occurs.

You can customize a cooking therapy session to target an emotional or mental health issue or to use a particular food, meal, or setting. In other words, a cooking therapy session can be created inside out (emotion) or outside in (setting or ingredients).

When you think about cooking therapy, remember, it's always available and ready for you. Every time you prepare a meal or snack, there is the opportunity to mine the food prep for a mini or major clinical result. If you are whipping up a recipe that calls for ten ingredients, you can look up those ingredients beforehand and have ten different personalized prompts to incorporate immediately into your meal preparation. The personalized cooking therapy combinations will be different each time, depending on the recipe you prepare.

The Al Dente Rules of a Cooking Therapy Session

I have a few simple rules that ensure you will get the most out of cooking therapy. Read through these all the way, and then feel free to reference this list whenever you need to. By staying in the present moment and embracing the process, you're sure to have a terrific session.

1. **First, stay totally focused on the therapy session.** To do this, intentionally carve out the necessary time, limit distractions, put away cell phones and tablets, and give yourself the gift of the allotted time just as if you were in a therapist's office. If you value the session this way, it will pay more dividends. Take a moment or two to remind yourself that this is a strategic and clinical session. Remind yourself that you are not just cooking but engaging in cooking therapy and it will require you to use the 3M curriculum. You will be mindful; tease out metaphors to reflect self-talk, feelings, and behaviors; and incorporate small and large moments of mastery that will infuse you with self-applause.

2. **Next, name your recipes.** Starting in Chapter 6 of the book, I will do it for you, but when you create your own session recipes, it's essential that you give them a name that is accurate and positive. First, think about what you're going to address. Is it a situation that is stressing you out? Then work relieving stress into the name of your recipe. A soup could become "Settle Down Soup," or a brownie recipe could be named "Becoming Balanced Brownies." Start with your dish, then add the relevant title. Have some fun with it and remember that this applies to every dish, even if it's just a salad or a sandwich. A salad that is called "Fresh Outlook Greens" will remind you that you were searching for another way to view a situation. If you only say, "I

made a salad," it's not likely to stick after the session ends. Just saying "I made a sandwich" will probably not remind you of anything later. But "The Layers of Me Sandwich" surely will.

3. **Always "take stock" of your "ingredients."** These are the thoughts and emotions that are inside you at the start of the session. What are you bringing to the table today? Optimism? Exhaustion? Hope? It's important to know. In a therapist's office, the first question is likely to be "What's going on?" Or "How can I help you today?" I subscribe to the tenet that "the therapy begins with the first phone call." You know that when you first contact a therapist, you begin to think about why in a more concrete way. Give yourself that same gift. By tapping into your feelings first, you can maximize the work and the benefit.

To access those feelings, stand at the counter, place both hands at your sides, and name two feelings you're experiencing. You needn't close your eyes, just focus. Now, rate them in your mind on a scale of one to five, with one being the weakest and five being most intense. This will put you in an active state, as a participant in your own journey, rather than simply a vessel to collect information. Think of therapy as fluid. It's a moving process. And how you participate is crucial to progress. There is discovering to determine discovery, revealing to create a revelation. Now, take a deep breath. Recommit to being a participant, and get ready for the next steps. If you practice and integrate the process of tapping into your feelings and thoughts, you will gain the skills to make self-awareness a habit rather than a goal.

Once again, be present. This means you commit to doing more than cooking; you commit to participating in cooking therapy. I think of being present as a verb, an action verb, rather than a noun. This is the beginning of the CBT process. Identify your thoughts, evaluate them for veracity, experiment with new ones, and assess the change. While there is much Zen to be found in cooking, clinical progress begins with being mindful that this is a purposeful and therapeutic experience. When simply cooking, you can multitask or zone out and still be enjoying the experience. In cooking therapy, I want you zoned in on your thoughts, your patterns, and the feelings attached to them.

4. **Next, practice *mise en place*.** Translated from French, it means "putting everything in its place." This is the term for getting everything prepped to be cooked as the orders come in. It's precise and comprehensive—vegetables chopped, broth simmering, spices measured, all in the service of the food being cooked perfectly and the meals being served tout de suite (quickly ☺). When we say "mise en place" purposefully at the start of a session, it has a way of binding us or readying us to begin. Before a cooking therapy session, read the recipes to know what ingredients or appliances you will need. Put them in place; it will make it easier to be focused during the session. Gather any measuring cups or spoons, bowls, utensils, and ingredients and place them on your counter or table, even if you're just creating a bowl of cereal or a dish of ice cream.

There is one time when we divert from mise en place, and that is when it comes to having everything "in place" about what we're feeling or knowing. The beauty of a session is that we don't have everything "chopped perfectly" or "seasoned correctly" in our thoughts and emotions. We have room for mess and change and movement and mistakes! So be ready to go, but don't worry if you're ambivalent, unsure, or even unmoored without knowing exactly why. Bring your insecurities and imperfections and questions. Unlike the dishes or orders in a Michelin-starred restaurant, there is no pressure to "cook yourself perfectly." Emotionally, just show up, because everyone has a prime table at this establishment.

5. **Speaking of mistakes,** *there are none*! Why? Once again, Cooking therapy is always about the process and not the result. You may question how a session without a traditional success can produce mastery. The mastery in cooking therapy, like any therapy session, is that you showed up and did the work. Even more, if you've learned something, uncovered something about yourself, or had a realization such as *Oh, I've never thought of it that way before*, then you've truly mastered getting to know yourself or your patterns. The results are not always what you see in front of you and may appear later. If you've been in traditional therapy, you know that sometimes a moment from the session becomes clear to you in the future, often when you're about to repeat a pattern. Here are some examples of "mistakes" that are not mistakes and can be reframed:

- The bread didn't rise? Perhaps we have made pitas, crackers, or breadcrumbs.
- Cream overwhipped? We've got butter!

- Rice too sticky? Rinse with warm water, and let's "unstick" other things.
- Lumps in a sauce or gravy? Pulverize and contemplate "taking your lumps."
- Salmon or shrimp overcooked? Let's add to a salad, wrap, or taco.

6. **Finally, always wash your hands before you begin.** Yes, it's hygienic, but it's also a metaphor for beginning and for a fresh start or idea. It's a tangible decision to begin with a clean outlook and mindset, unmuddied by old thoughts and behaviors. It may seem a small moment, but cooking therapy is made up of many such small moments that come together for a big impact, from noticing, mining the process for metaphors, and achievement. Or, as I've already told you, mindfulness, metaphors, and mastery!

Now that you have an understanding of what cooking therapy is, it's time to uncover the power of what it does with cooking therapy sessions that will empower and infuse you with calm, clarity, and confidence. Let's get started.

PART 2

Cooking Therapy Your Way

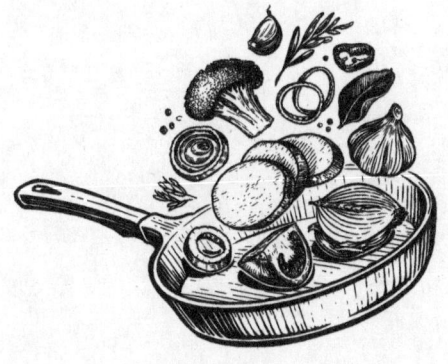

Chapter Six

Session One: Creating Calm

A recipe has no soul. You, as the cook, must bring soul to the recipe.

—Thomas Keller

A few years ago, I worked with a ten-year-old girl who was sleep-deprived from her fears and worries. This was creating consequences in school and even with friendships. Her personality was changing due to the constant exhaustion and anxiety. Her parents had tried everything, from monitoring and limiting TV time to nightly rituals of checking her room for monsters. A frequent complaint she had was that terrorists could be hiding under her bed. Even with checking, she remained unconvinced. Though she was naming something specific, fear of terrorists, I felt it was more likely that an overall feeling of insecurity and lack of safety was driving the fears. A picture she drew of her family showed her parents and older brother all the same size, but her figure was much, much taller than anyone. This represented to me her feeling too adult or responsible for her age.

This was in no way the family's doing. The girl's mom and dad were nurturing and involved. If anything, they gave her almost too much attention, which may have inadvertently contributed to her sense that she was needy. Sadly, I believe this is an example of the uncertainty many young people—and adults too—feel today. Uncertainty can be processed by some with no consequence, and yet for others it can be unnerving.

I cooked with my young client to create a sense of calm and peace, naming the recipe "Calming Cookies." We took a lot of delicious breaths, and not only were the smells soothing, but it was an opportunity to teach breathing techniques.

If you're feeling a bit unmoored or frenetic, then I hope the recipes that follow will help and that you'll be able to integrate more peace, calm, and balance into your daily life.

When it comes to creating calm, I encourage you to create a space that supports peace and beauty. You don't need a fancy kitchen or chef-level utensils. Pick some fresh flowers, buy a pretty mug, plate your food with intention. After cooking, think about safely lighting some candles that appeal to your senses. Ocean breeze and florals in spring and summer and vanilla or cinnamon in the autumn or winter? It's up to you. If you surround yourself and appeal to your senses with things you value and that inspire you, you will feel worthy and elevated. Pretty simple. When it comes to plating, especially, the metaphor is clear; you've put so much time and effort into the session, and a little thought about the beauty and balance of it will help to cement the great work you've done.

As always, in each session, remember to:

1. Respect the space
2. Name the recipe (I've done it here for you)
3. Take stock of what you've brought to the table
4. Be present
5. Wash your hands before you begin

FAST LANE: Brightening Balance Bread

You're about to start your day or you have a few minutes at another time and you're feeling a bit stressed, so you'd like to infuse a quick therapy session into your day? You've come to the right place. This is one of the miracles of cooking therapy, the double-duty bonus, breakfast with a side of serenity. Today in the Fast Lane, we'll be making "Brightening Balance Bread."

Ingredients

2 slices of bread, any kind; an English muffin; or a bagel

2 tablespoons soft butter, margarine, cream cheese, jelly, or jam

Session Instructions

1. Turn on the toaster oven. Heat is a catalyst for change. As you turn the toaster on, acknowledge that you are going to try to make a change by infusing a new feeling of calm into your day.
2. Remove the bread from its package and take a moment to notice the smell of freshness. Take slow, deep breaths and let it fill your senses.
3. Notice that the bread or bagel has holes or pockets. Take a moment to visualize "emptying your pockets" of items that are stressing you out. Then imagine refilling those pockets with new objects, like calm, peace, and harmony.
4. Toast the bread and imagine warming up to the idea of not taking in the stress as you have in the past. Feel the

warmth of the toaster and your bread and let that sink in. Stay with it a few seconds.

5. Spread the butter or jam of your choice purposefully. You are tangibly adding a softness, sweetness, and smoothness to your mood with purpose and intent.

6. Take a bite; notice the taste and texture. If you feel stressed later, try to recreate the moment you feel right now.

TO GO

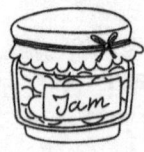 As you eat your breakfast or snack and, later, process the session by remembering the steps, recall two moments of mindfulness in the session to use as needed in the future. Here are some questions to ask yourself:

- Does the idea of heating up inspire you to think about a new attitude?
- Visualize emptying your pockets of stress and filling them with calm.
- What about the actual smell of freshness? How does that resonate and motivate you to breathe differently?

Though it was a short session, once you have completed the recipe, if you felt calmer, resolve to cement this feeling of mindful mastery for later. At the end of the day, reflect on whether you can internalize the session to spread a buttery softness into your mood and day.

EASY RIDER: Feeling Brand Newdles

If you have about an hour to spend and you'd like to feel lighter by preparing a recipe that's less rushed than the Fast Lane, then zoodles or noodles are for you. You're going to feel different and less stressed with "Feeling Brand Newdles."

Ingredients

For the noodles

1 container spiralized zoodles or ½ pound noodles/ long pasta
½ cucumber
1 pint cherry tomatoes

½ red onion, sliced or chopped
½ yellow or orange bell pepper
Crumbled feta cheese; may substitute to taste

For the dressing

2 tablespoons extra-virgin olive oil
2 tablespoons lemon juice

1 teaspoon oregano
Salt and pepper to taste

Session Instructions

1. If you're cooking noodles, cook them according to the package directions. If you're using zoodles, skip to step five. Think of something that makes you "boiling mad."
2. Prepare a very large bowl with ice water and place it in the sink. Place a colander next to it in the sink.
3. When the pasta is ready, pour it into the colander, lift the colander, and plunge it into the bowl of ice water.

Hold your face directly over the bowl as the steam dissipates and think of letting go of anything that makes you "steamy." The next time you feel boiling mad, REMEMBER this moment and "bring down the heat."

4. Lift the colander and let the noodles "drain," just as if you were letting your anger or frustration or tension drain away. Once again, think about going from "overheated" to cool and letting tension drain away.

5. Separate the zoodles or noodles, and as you do, notice the strands. They look like nerves, all wound up and tangled, a perfect visual of stress! Set your intent. You're going to pull the strands apart and loosen them, and while you're doing so, imagine doing the same with the retes of nerves in your mind. Soften the stress and transform it into a smoother, less tangled state.

6. Now let's peel the cucumbers. Think about any part of your life that is dark and bitter and peel back to get an honest look. Maybe you'll even peel away some negativity from family dynamics, work situations, or challenging friends. Perhaps you've simply been perfectionistic or "hard" on yourself in some way. As the dark green disappears, what do you see? Lightness? Coolness? Maybe even some seeds of change? Take a mindful moment or two to let it stay with you.

7. Chop the cucumbers into bite-size, "manageable" bites. It's always easier to reduce stress when you break it down into one or two items. Bite size is always more manageable than chunks. It's very hard to tackle a gigantic, unclear, and overwhelming sense of tension. Each time you make a cut, think to yourself *Little by little, I can identify a source and make small changes.* Once you do, plan to breathe through it or

communicate a different way, or even just decide to let it go and laugh more. Only you can decide. I know it seems like a light fix, but it works. One bite at a time. Then take a moment to think about what you want to "cut into your life" or change.

8. Tomatoes have come to represent change for me, as their insides are filled with seeds and a kind of gel, as if they were picked before they were finished growing. And you, no matter how old you are, just like these tomatoes, aren't done growing; you're still evolving. Halve the tomatoes; look at the gelatinous inside of one half as how you feel now and let the other half represent a change you've always wanted to make. Take a moment to really think about how your "other half" might change. What would provide more tranquility in your life? Meditation? Travel? More family time? *Less* family time ☺? Crystallizing what's missing can be the first step in adding to the salad that is you. You're not "done," so think about one small thing you can do going forward to add to your joy, which I promise will convert to inner stillness.

9. Olives are oily and tangy and add flavor. They are not the main dish; they are the something-something that can add a tang. First, have perspective. You cannot be calm and balanced all the time. Accept the "tangy" days. Then think about the olive pits. Sometimes "secrets" are a cause for stress. The olives are pitted, and you may want to acknowledge any secrets that leave you with that "pit" inside. Not all secrets should be shared, but this is a good time to examine whether yours are helping or hurting.

10. Onions can represent things that make us cry. Slicing or chopping a red onion does that to most people.

Crying can be good, but holding everything in? Not so much. Let yourself mourn or grieve the things that have contributed to anger, sadness, frustration, words unsaid, or moves not made.

11. Chop the peppers into large or small pieces. This part is up to you and taps into your own creativity and self-image. We will be adding them for color and balance, so you decide the size that best represents who you are or want to be. Visual appeal can be its own metaphor in cooking therapy. Prior to adding the peppers we have the colors green and red; now we add a new color to represent newness and beauty near the end of the session. You'll be surprised at how small moments of beauty or color can calm. Take a moment to enjoy the colors.

12. Finally, sprinkle the crumbled cheese on top and throughout. This metaphor is one of my favorites. Sprinkling goodness into the salad is like sprinkling goodness into your life. If you consciously sprinkle more compliments, gratitude, and blessings into the world, they will come back to you as deliciously as the cheese will taste to you in this salad.

13. Mix the dressing ingredients together and contemplate mixing together everything you've just done and learned.

14. Add the dressing and toss. Let the salad soak up the dressing as you soak up a mindful and masterful moment of enjoying your "Feeling Brand Newdles." Eat it right away or chill it in the refrigerator until it's ready to eat. This can act as a metaphor not to act impulsively. Next time you think about lashing out, especially to yourself, remember to "let it rest" or chill.

TO GO

Process the session by remembering how you brought down the heat with the noodles. Internalize that metaphor for something going on in your life. Imagine draining any negative emotions you may encounter during the day. Also think about how you loosened strands that were tight and that were reminiscent of stress, and imagine doing the same on your own. Here are some questions to ask yourself:

- Think about peeling away darkness to uncover the lightness and freshness in yourself underneath.
- Identify at least one "piece" of stress you can attack as a bite and how you can evolve, or are evolving, like the tomato.
- Ask what you can sprinkle into your day to improve it. Thanks? Blessings? Gratitude?

If you felt a sense of accomplishment after completing the recipe, cement this feeling of mastery for later.

SCENIC DRIVE: Moderate Your Mood Meatloaf

I'm a big fan of meatloaf, because it's comforting to make and a comfort food. This recipe is both sweet and tangy, which is an awful lot like most of us. I've used this recipe to "spice up" a "stale" marriage but also to sweeten the mood for individuals and couples. Feel free to be creative and customize "Moderate Your Mood Meatloaf" to taste. In fact, studies show that creativity diminishes stress.

Ingredients

For the meatloaf

1 pound ground meat; can be
   beef, turkey, or lamb or a
   combination
1 cup breadcrumbs or panko
1 egg

½ cup sweetened applesauce
2 teaspoons whole-grain
   mustard
Dash of salt and pepper

For the filling

½ cup sweetened
   applesauce
1 tablespoon brown sugar

1 tablespoon vinegar
1 tablespoon Dijon mustard

Session Instructions

1. Preheat your oven to 350 degrees. Always think of heat
   as a catalyst for change. Your dish will change from
   "raw" to "baked," and as it changes, so can you.

2. Remove the meat from the refrigerator and place it in a
   large bowl. Let it sit on the counter for a bit. We want
   the coldness to ease so the meat is easier to handle
   with your hands. "Easier to handle" is your first metaphor. If you feel that your sense of calm or worry is
   excessive and causing constant "freezing," then you
   may be experiencing generalized anxiety disorder
   and/or panic attacks, which can be treated. See the
   note at the end of the recipe.

3. Add the crumbs to the meat, focusing on the word *crumbs*
   for two reasons: First, you always deserve more than
   crumbs in life. Second, just in case you feel like crumbling
   sometimes, remind yourself that you can add strength
   and build yourself back up, just as the crumbs added to
   the meat will make a solid foundation for the loaf.

4. Crack the egg into the mixture and think of "birthing" a new change into your life. Think of the egg coming into the mixture (you) and pouring a new and original way to feel. Now, add the applesauce and whole-grain mustard into the mix to represent that life is both sweet and sour at times—and that's okay.

5. Mix these ingredients together with your hands. It will feel sticky. As you mix, do so mindfully, imagining that you're creating a new way of feeling and thinking. You are the one that shapes how you feel, no matter what others may do. The mixing may also feel like hard work, but that's often how it is when you feel stressed or pressured. But with hard work there's some pride and ownership too, right? You're not sitting around waiting for change to magically occur, you're actively doing something. As you accomplish this, it will be exponentially effective in all areas of your life.

6. In a square pan, shape the mixture into a round loaf. Sounds like that expression *square peg in a round hole*, but actually it's the opposite. A square peg does not fit in a round hole, but a round shape will fit nicely in a square pan, and that's a representation that change can happen. It will look like a circle in a square. Tell yourself you are shaping a new attitude with fewer or no sharp edges.

7. Now take the back of a spoon and make a round depression in the top of the loaf where the filling will go. I hate to use the word depression in a mood changing session, and we could substitute the word crater if you like, but we can smile about this together, too. I told you Cooking therapy would also be fun, right? And smacking that spoon into the meat makes a wonderful "be gone stress" sound. Enjoy it.

8. Mix the filling ingredients together, noting that while the vinegar and mustard are more closely related to sharpness, which represents anxiety, there is a greater amount of applesauce and brown sugar, which will turn the sharp into the sweet. Please name two things that are sweet in your life. Don't just do that in the session. "Smack them" into your brain all the time. I promise you this will help and will be part of your emotional tool kit long term.

9. Fill the crater with the filling. Now emphasize to yourself that you are doing something tangible and concrete to *fill* yourself with stillness.

10. Bake the loaf for an hour or until cooked through, until the internal temperature is 160°F. During this time, activate all your senses and especially your sense of accomplishment. You've cooked through an amazing cooking therapy session. Perhaps you can retrieve your phone (just this once) and take a photo! Serve your "Moderate Your Mood Meatloaf" right away or let it rest; the choice is yours. When you slice it and serve it, think about slicing in your new skills and serving up self-applause.

TO GO

Remember that you worked to mix up a new feeling, and going forward, try to remember the power of shaping your intent for calm. Here are some prompts and reminders to take with you:

- It's possible to add more sweetness than sour.
- Remember that you can fill yourself or others with goodness and also that all of the acts of shaping,

filling, or smacking are intended to give you the power to change your mood.

- Remember, too, the moments of mindfulness in this session.
- When you feel anxious in the future, think about finding things to fill yourself up, like you did with the crater, and do not accept crumbs!

Note: Generalized anxiety disorder and panic attacks are two recognized conditions that are frequently treated by therapists. For more information, see the Resources section (page 259) at the end of the book.

After-Dinner Mint

Remember, most traditional therapy sessions do not create breakthroughs in one session but rather after rapport has been established, comfort has been reached, and some of the thoughts and questions have had time to "marinate." This can happen days, weeks, and months later.

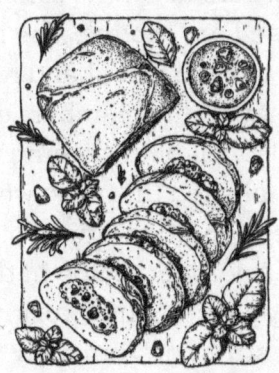

Chapter Seven

Session Two: Infusing Confidence

The only real stumbling block is fear of failure. In cooking, you've got to have a what-the-hell attitude.

—Julia Child

Like many teenage girls, Sophie, a sophomore in high school, was struggling with poor self-esteem. Sophie was smart, pretty, athletic, and very friendly and polite. Despite this, she saw herself as awkward and "less than" some of the "popular" girls at school. In our work together, we focused on her self-esteem issues.

One of my favorite techniques with both children and adults is the "Post-it" technique. The client takes a full pack of small Post-its and writes an appropriate affirming phrase on each one, then puts them everywhere so that they see the phrase all day. This means placing Post-its in all the rooms in the house, outside, in the car, in schoolbooks, etc. For Sophie, we chose *I am enough!* The impact of this technique is in the bombardment and repetition. And it doesn't hurt the other family members either. Sophie's mom reported that she also felt better seeing the affirmations.

Once we accomplished this task, we decided to create a cooking therapy session titled "I've Got the Stuff Stuffing," which will be the Easy Rider recipe in this chapter. I used it as a chance for Sophie to name positive attributes and create her own self-stuffing. Ultimately we mined the metaphor for "stuff I'm made of" and "stuff I'd like to add over time."

It's amazing how audiovisuals can play an important part in any emotional journey. *Moomba* is a motivational acronym that stands for "my only obstacle is my bad attitude" or "my only obstacle may be attitude." The best part about a Moomba is that it's meant to be shared as a tangible good and placed in a spot that is viewed often (similar to the Post-its discussed earlier). Mine is a piece of red yarn that was given to me by one of my supervisors with the message to pay it forward. It hangs on my makeup mirror. I've given Moombas made of string or cloth, and I know one therapist who has had a rubber bracelet made with the word *Moomba* on it. She wears it daily.

Remember this story as you engage in every cooking therapy session. You will listen to the lessons and hear the metaphors, but you will also visualize how clarity and change happen.

As always, in each session remember to:

1. Respect the space
2. Name the recipe (I've done it here for you)
3. Take stock of what you've brought to the table
4. Be present
5. Wash your hands before you begin

FAST LANE: You Are Most Certainly Superb Cereal

Short on time but need a little infusion of self-worth? You'll find it here with a simple serving of "You Are Most

Certainly Superb Cereal." You can make this dish with any cereal of your choice. You can use any type of milk, such as almond, oat, or dairy milk with any level of fat.

Ingredients

¾ cup cereal of your choice

¾ cup milk of your choice

½ cup berries, fruit, or nuts

Session Instructions

1. Shake the box of cereal. Take a mindful moment to notice the noise. Guess what? That's applause. For you. For all the things you've done right and well or with good intentions that you forgot to congratulate yourself about. Take a minute to remember one specific accomplishment and praise yourself.

2. Pour the cereal into a bowl. Think of pouring affirmations into yourself. What kinds of things can you say to start the day or simply build yourself up? How about "I appreciate myself"? Or "I choose to like myself?" Or perhaps you have a challenge ahead. As you pour the cereal, pour confidence and say out loud, "I can do it."

3. Pour the milk onto the cereal. How does it look? Smooth, cool, creamy, flowing? *All* good ways to feel about yourself and the day ahead or behind you.

4. Notice the slight or big ways the milk changes color. Change is always possible. If you've had negative self-talk, this is a great time to alter the dialogue between you and you.

5. Choose a topping. The word *topping* is your cue to "top off all your good thoughts" and to tell yourself ... wait for it ... yes, you will come out on top, and you are tops!

Ahhh, semantics are a gift in cooking therapy. Use them often. Don't diminish the power. Say it again as you eat, even if you're in a rush. "I'll come out on top. I am tops."

TO GO

Continue to pour positive thoughts, change if you'd like to, keep cool, and tell yourself often that you're tops. Here are some reminders as you take this session with you:

- Sometimes it helps to write down two of the steps that were most impactful and any metaphor that worked for you.
- Don't forget to applaud yourself frequently and cement the feeling of accomplishment so you can use it as needed.

The next time you feel yourself becoming envious of others or tough on yourself, please revisit this goody bag.

EASY RIDER: I've Got the Stuff Stuffing

Earlier in this chapter I told you about Sophie and her stuff. I talk a lot about "stuff" in this book. It's not a clinical term, is it? But it's become colloquial for so many of us and shows up in lots of clichés. *She's carrying a lot of stuff. He's hot stuff. Show off your stuff. You need tougher stuff.* Endless. Well, I'm not actually a fan of clichés, but I can't help myself; it's just too perfect for this recipe. In "I've Got the Stuff Stuffing," I use a bag of store-bought, already-seasoned stuffing cubes, but if you've got loads of time, feel free to use fresh bread.

Ingredients

2 tablespoons butter or margarine

Enough celery for ½ cup chopped

Enough onion for ½ cup chopped

2 tablespoons chopped sage

3¹/³ cups water or chicken broth

1 ½-ounce package seasoned stuffing mix (or approximately 16 slices of bread)

> Note: If using fresh bread, you will need stuffing seasoning (combine 2 teaspoons salt, 1 teaspoon paprika, and 1/3 cup chopped parsley)

Session Instructions

1. Melt the butter in a large saucepan over medium heat. Melting is the beginning step for infusing. You need something to infuse into, right? Think of the butter as the part of you that hasn't been ready to take in the assurances that you have the right stuff and that you are enough, just the way you are. Medium heat feels just right for doing things moderately in a way that will make everything come together without boring you to death or, worse, burning you out.

2. Chop the celery and onion. Sometimes putting things into little pieces can represent making big problems little, but here I want you to focus on the chopping. Not in anger, but to think about chopping in all the individual ingredients you already have that make your stuff enough stuff. In addition, perhaps there are some attributes you aspire to, like compassion or self-reliance or

individuality. If you're aspiring to obtain more or different attributes, here is a chance to think about getting those traits ready to be incorporated.

3. Add the celery and onion to the pan and cook till they soften. This should take three to five minutes, enough time for you to name three things you're good at. Here's a hint: something you do or something you are. Go!

4. Mix in the chopped sage. Sage is the perfect ingredient for focusing on wise choices, aka "sage advice." While you may be "enough," there is always room to examine your choices and commit to thoughtful and smart behaviors. In your mind, commit to giving thorough thought rather than snap decisions when it comes to future endeavors.

5. Add the broth and seasoning, either the packet from the box or the stuffing seasoning, if you're using fresh bread. Think of the broth as your base. It's going to work two ways: First, it's going to absorb whatever you put into it, and it's going to infuse *into* those same items. Stop and think for a second moment to cement the idea of infusion; if the base is you, what qualities do you want to acquire, and what do you already have? Seasonings you want, seasonings you have. These are traits. For example, for confidence, you may already have a friendly nature but be hesitant to speak first. You may be smart or creative or funny as hell but unsure of how to share those qualities with the world. Often, fear is a big factor. That's kind of like the broth. It's mild, but when you add seasoning, it may be spicy or tangy. Guess what? It tastes great with seasoning! Learn to like "your seasoning," and you will learn to like yourself. Also, sometimes we may overseason or underseason, and that's okay. If "overseasoning" happens in life, add a little something else like patience or explanation. If you

feel it's the opposite, "underseason," just add more, like embracing your personality and sharing it.

6. If using fresh bread, trim the crusts. What a perfect metaphor for removing any hard or "crusty" parts or old attitudes! Then cut them into cubes. If using the bag of cubes, you'll notice they are hard, so we'll be softening these too. Add them to the saucepan and toss lightly. It's a light toss of new ideas and behaviors into old ones.

7. Preheat the oven to 350 degrees. Think about the oven getting ready to receive your new ideas and seal them into a solid start. Place the stuffing mixture into a 9 × 13 pan or glass dish like Pyrex. If the mixture looks too flat, use a slightly smaller dish like 8 × 8. And that's a lot like life and confidence. Sometimes we overstep and have to pull back. At other times we reach too far and must temper our goals. But we never stop putting ourselves "into the dish."

8. Once the oven is preheated, bake for 30 minutes or until the top looks slightly browned. Take a long look at your stuffing. Notice how delicious it smells. Don't just let it cool and walk away. Stare at it; share with someone if possible. It's a dish of mastery and confidence that you created and will remind you that "you've got the stuff."

TO GO

Here are some important reminders as you work on mastery:

- Remember that you're already full of "seasonings," traits that work for you and those you can adjust.
- Toss new ideas lightly and remove hard crusts.
- Don't forget to melt a little to infuse positivity.

- Take a moment to say out loud a few ways that you'll "overseason" or "underseason" in real life, and when you do, try to write down how it went.
- Sometimes putting things down on paper can crystallize results.
- No matter what happens, say out loud three times, "I've got the stuff!"
- If you were insecure about something, how did you feel before you began, and how do you feel now?

The next time you feel yourself becoming insecure, afraid, or hesitant to try new things or be yourself, refer to this section and remind yourself that you've got the stuff.

SCENIC DRIVE: You Are Estellar Brownies, Times 2

Part of the paralyzing self-doubt some of us feel comes from our own negative self-talk. In this way we make confidence more elusive and harder to obtain. As a young girl, I helped my mother make brownies to send to my brother, who was overseas in the Army. It was an arduous task. We had no KitchenAids or Cuisinarts or any fancy appliances, and without electronics, the most difficult part of making that recipe was creaming the butter and sugar together until the mixture was smooth and there were no granules. As a child, my arm would eventually ache.

That same recipe my mom and I made those years ago has now turned into the recipe below, "You are Estellar Brownies, Times 2." My mom's name was Estelle, so I've named this recipe in her honor. This recipe showcases the way we make things harder or easier for ourselves, and the metaphor is meant to model the difference between easy and hard. Many of us tend to make things hard on ourselves when it isn't necessary. Consciously deciding not to do that will become easier if you follow these instructions.

If you were doing this recipe the hard way, it would be with elbow grease, sometimes known as pain! You would grease and flour two pans with softened butter and flour, not baking spray. There would be no microwave, so you would have had to plan early, leaving the butter out to soften. Using the back of a spoon, you would cream together butter and sugar till smooth. By the time this was done, you may have needed to ice your sore arm.

Next, you would melt the chocolate in the top of a double boiler. No microwave.

You would then add eggs one at a time, mixing after each. Then mix in the flour and vanilla and pour into the two pans. A lot of work, right?

But, luckily, together we are simply going to make our brownies with all of our modern conveniences. This is a stark and powerful reminder to stop doubting yourself and remember that you always have a choice. Each time you default to being difficult with yourself, remember this recipe, and you will be easier on yourself.

Ingredients

1 cup butter, unsalted (softened, not melted)

Baking spray or extra butter for greasing pan

2 cups sugar

4 squares unsweetened chocolate, melted

4 eggs

1 cup flour, self-rising, extra for greasing pan

1 teaspoon vanilla

Session Instructions

1. Preheat the oven to 350 degrees. Remember that heat signifies change. I'd like you to make a commitment right now to truly entertaining a new way to talk to yourself. As your oven gets warm, think about speaking more warmly to yourself.

2. Butter the pan or spray it with cooking spray, then flour it, which will make everything so much easier, with no mess, and think about clearing out any messy thoughts. These are the ones that make you doubt yourself or minimize your achievements.

3. Combine softened butter and sugar using a paddle attachment in an electric bowl stand (like a KitchenAid) or an electric hand mixer. Keep the mixer stirring on medium for about three to four minutes until the mixture is lighter and fluffier and a pale-yellow color. Blend in positive thoughts. Remember that achievements don't have to be like climbing Mount Everest or winning an Olympic gold medal. Sometimes just getting through a tough day at work or getting the kids dressed and off to school is enough, and it should fill you with a sense of accomplishment.

4. In a small bowl, melt the chocolate for approximately thirty seconds in the microwave, and add it to the bowl with the sugar-and-butter mixture. Once again, as the seconds tick off, melt away any remaining negative thoughts.

5. Add the eggs to the bowl one at a time. As you crack each egg, invite optimism into yourself and empty any pessimism from your mind.

6. Measure out sifted, self-rising flour and gradually add it to the bowl. Physically stand up on your tiptoes with

your arms stretched up and imagine yourself rising up out of disappointments. Then sift through the thoughts that may be keeping you down. Dump them!

7. Add vanilla and think of yourself as multilayered and colorful. Name two of these layers of you or things that are bright about you and say them out loud.

8. Add the batter to the greased and floured pan and bake for thirty minutes or until a toothpick comes out clean. During the baking time, sit with all your positive thoughts. Remove the pan from the oven, and as the brownies cool and come together, let all of the positive self-talk steps in this recipe gel.

TO GO

When the brownies are done and cooled, reflect. How long might the difficult method have taken compared to our modern and fairly easy method? They may have both looked and tasted the same, but you know that being harder on yourself is never necessary and taking it easy on yourself can be a conscious and delicious choice. Here are some ideas to marinate on:

- It may be helpful to write down two of the steps that were most impactful and why as well as a particular metaphor that worked for you and explain why.
- Can you name two ways you'll remember to be easier on yourself and cement the feeling of mastery for later?
- It may be helpful to use a Likert scale to assess how you felt before and after a session. On a scale of one to five, with five being very tough on yourself, how did you feel before you began and how do you feel now?

The next time you feel yourself becoming envious of others or tough on yourself, refer back to this section and remind yourself that even though we only made these brownies one easy way, you are "Estellar," times two!

After-Dinner Mint

Remember, most traditional therapy sessions do not create breakthroughs in one session but rather after rapport has been established, comfort has been reached, and some of the thoughts and questions have had time to "marinate." This can happen days, weeks, and months later.

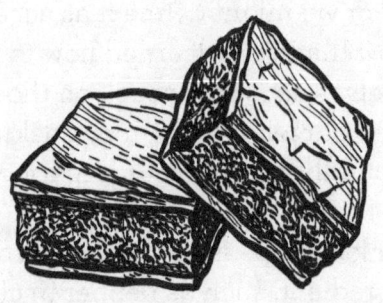

Chapter Eight

Session Three: Radical Self-Acceptance

Food is not about impressing people. It's about making them feel comfortable.

—Ina Garten

Radical acceptance is a term we take from DBT (dialectical behavior therapy) to describe accepting things in the world as they are. Many of us simplify this sentiment by saying, "It is what it is," or we might define it as accepting "life on life's terms." Now that we've learned how to infuse confidence into ourselves, let's piggyback on those lessons and learn to empower ourselves even more, asking whether it is possible to not only admit to our imperfections but to embrace them.

I always think a recipe is more interesting when it has a surprising ingredient, such as pepper in chocolate. Have you tried beer can chicken or baked apples with cherry soda? These dishes celebrate a unique method or ingredient. In beer can chicken, the whole bird is cooked standing up on an open beer can. The liquid tenderizes the chicken while infusing it with an unexpected flavor.

For the apples dish, baked apples are cored and placed whole into a baking dish, then doused in cherry or black cherry soda. The same principle applies here, as we are infusing, softening, and flavoring in a totally different way.

I've made a keto recipe where cauliflower and cashews come together to make you swear you're eating cheese-cake. The point is, instead of striving to be the "popular" dish, go for quirky and original; be you.

When you share your mishaps and doubts, others generally respond with kindness and connection. Every-one feels flawed to a certain extent, and it's freeing and comforting to know that you are not alone. Here is where the real friendships and relationships take root, in honest revelation.

Think of the powerful impact it would have on our confidence and satisfaction if we didn't always try so hard to prove to the world that we're doing great. Think of the radical internal relief! What would happen if each of us decided to create a press release to tell the world we're okay with ourselves, flaws and all. It could look something like this:

Sara S. Embraces Whole Personality

January 1, 2025: **In a shocking diversion from her usual need to promote perfection, Sara S. no longer wants to present a false picture to the world and vows to embrace her personality as a whole and like herself just the way she is.**

Embracing your whole personality might take some work, I know. It may not be what you're used to, but the recipes in the following chapter will help. None of them aspire to be fancy. None of them insist on the finest butter from France or expensive items like vanilla beans from Madagascar. But all of them will taste great, and that's the point. You don't have to look great for the world, just taste great to yourself.

I want to be überclear about radical acceptance. It isn't a study in sad acknowledgment, like a recipe gone bad, it's a joyful celebration of what is, like an unexpected but still oh-so-tasty dish.

The art of kintsugi is a wonderful Japanese method for repairing broken bowls and other objects. The philosophy of kintsugi is that the cracks and imperfections in broken items make them more beautiful, and so they are not repaired seamlessly. Instead, the fractures and flaws are illuminated with gold or silver paint. The artist actually embraces the objects and tries to get a sense of them before the breaks. He doesn't whitewash the objects and try to fix them perfectly or pretend the crevices never existed.

This is a powerful message we can extrapolate for ourselves and for integrating radical acceptance. Our imperfections are what they are and make us even more beautiful. Another example of CBT at work: When we change the way we think, we change the way we feel, and new behaviors follow.

As always, in each session remember to:

1. Respect the space
2. Name the recipe (I've done it here for you)
3. Take stock of what you've brought to the table
4. Be present
5. Wash your hands before you begin

FAST LANE: It's Never All Smooth Smoothie

Ahhh, the myth of the perfectly smooth life. Part urban legend, mostly a mirage, and just as elusive; every time you think you're there, it dissipates. As we now know, craving the perfect pot of gold is senseless and sometimes harmful to our self-concept. Most of us know in our heads and hearts that it doesn't exist. Instead, happiness is more likely determined by how we navigate the bumps; the smooth straightaways will take care of themselves. Enjoy them, but don't expect their permanence. Abide the tumbles and rolls. Let's cement our commitment to embracing imperfections with an easy and quick recipe for continuing resolve and the belief that "it's never all smooth." It's not a pot of gold, but still magically delicious.

You can substitute a wide variety of ingredients to make "It's Never All Smooth Smoothie." Just ensure that the ingredients *mirror the process* in each. Prefer mango to banana? Both are sweet, so that's fine. Coconut milk instead of yogurt? Soft and creamy, so sure. Kale or chard for spinach? They're both a little bitter and green, so that's fine too. You can even swap your protein powder for collagen, as they are both fortifying ingredients. Get the picture? Of course you do!

Ingredients

½ frozen banana
½ kiwi
½ cup each blueberries and
　　raspberries
½ cup yogurt of your choice

3–4 leaves spinach
1–2 scoops protein powder
Oats or chia seeds (optional)

Session Instructions

1. Place half a frozen banana in your blender. Think about starting your day without any hard feelings toward anyone. Make a commitment, at least for today, to cut through and pulverize any iciness you may feel. Remember the law of attraction? Direct warmth into the world, and less coldness comes back.

2. Kiwis have a hard and brown rind. Take a moment to think about how you present yourself to the world. Are you easy to get close to? Free with a smile or kind word? Peel the kiwi and think about what it would be like to go forward without a protective shell and be vulnerable and soft like the inside of a kiwi. Once it's peeled, chop it into small pieces and place in a bowl. Think about all the pieces of you and how you can make these small changes every day.

3. Wash the berries and place them in the bowl with the kiwi. Take a mindful moment to observe the colors. Gorgeous, right? Remind yourself that you have so many beautiful colors to you. Be still. Name three stunning inner attributes that make up who you are and say them out loud! Then add the kiwi and the berries to the mixer.

4. Spinach is not as sweet as the fruits but adds a dimension to the mix. What a perfect metaphor. We are not Suzy Sunshine all day long, and who would want to be? We are human and we can be slightly bitter or bland or even boring at times. Celebrate your humanity, add the leaves to the blender, and "leave" your need to be perpetually sweet out!

5. Spoon yogurt into the blender. How creamy and velvety would you like your day to be? Plan to achieve it as a

goal. As the day goes on, remember scooping this softness into the mixer and remind yourself to do the same with your attitude, your thoughts, and your actions.

6. The metaphor for protein powder is both obvious and powerful. Fortify yourself for whatever comes your way, today and, eventually, always. As you put the powder into the mix, acknowledge your strength and resolve to recall that no matter what happens, you are capable and competent.

7. Blend all the ingredients until smooth. Know that you've combined everything necessary for self-talk that allows you to befriend yourself, no matter how many bumps come your way. Let the noise of the mixer be a powerful and positive reminder that loud imperfections are okay. Once the smoothie is blended, pour your new way of thinking into a tall and "clear" glass. If you need an additional metaphor, top it with oats or seeds to remind you that bumps are not only okay but worthwhile.

TO GO

Remind yourself to embrace warmth instead of cold, open yourself up, notice beauty, accept all of your parts, keep cool, and celebrate the blend of all you are. Here are some questions to ask yourself as you process this session:

- Which of these steps or metaphors had the most impact on you, and which can you cement going forward?
- Try to feel less pressure to present yourself in a certain way, and if possible, write down two ways you'll accomplish this change.

- Remember that if you've had a need to appear flawless, it probably didn't serve you well and it may have even been intimidating to others. Most people don't mind a few bumps and bruises, because then they feel comfortable about their own.

Refer back to this process as needed and especially if at any time you feel yourself becoming envious of others or down on yourself.

EASY RIDER: Satisfied With Self Sandwich

There's a song by the musical group Train called "Bruises." In the song, a duet, the singers claim they want to fix each other. It's well intentioned, but then, in a moment of clarity and unison, they both agree not to fix anything about the other. They seem to realize that "fixing someone" is not a recipe for a healthy relationship.

When we begin to get comfortable with the idea of wearing and sharing our bruises, a world of acceptance and peace comes our way. In addition to being a therapist, I'm also an author and novelist, and I teach creative writing to seniors. These are folks in their eighties and nineties who have much to say and, as I've learned, even more to teach. Many of their responses to prompts and assignments astonish me, both in terms of creativity and wisdom. Some common themes include having no regrets, embracing a sense of humor about imperfections and mistakes, and letting shame and disappointments go. Imagine if we could learn this in our twenties, thirties, or forties!

Below is a recipe called "Satisfied With Self Sandwich," which will model the layers you can build on to establish self-acceptance and a resolve to abandon negativity.

Ingredients

1 bagel or 2 slices of bread
1–2 tablespoons mayonnaise
    or mustard
1–2 lettuce leaves (little gem
    if possible; iceberg or
    romaine will do)

1 slice onion
2 slices either turkey, ham,
    salami, or other meat
2 slices Swiss cheese

Session Instructions

1. Turn on your toaster or toaster oven. Think about heat and how it's a catalyst to change your current view or perspective.
2. Bread is often called the staff of life. Think about it as the basis for your life; it's who you are "on a plate." If you are using a bagel, slice it in half and think about slicing in all parts of you. If you are a "scooper," then scoop out damaging self-talk. If you are using bread, separate the slices from the loaf—at the same time separating feelings of negativity about your perceived flaws—and "open them up," readying them for new information.
3. Place the bread or bagel in the oven to warm and get ready to warm up to yourself more than you've done in the past.
4. When the bread/bagel is ready, remove it to a plate and spread with mayo or mustard. Set your intention for today and tomorrow. What are you going to spread into your day, your sense of self, your family life, and the world? It might be cool, creaminess, like the mayonnaise, or it might be a spicy bite, like the mustard. Either

is okay and both are needed at times. Both are a purposeful choice.

5. Now, as you layer your lettuce leaves, say out loud, "LET
   US" celebrate me! If you were able to get little gem
   lettuce, then remind yourself that you are a little gem
   and think about gems like diamonds; none are flawless,
   all sparkle. If you're using iceberg, then affirm that you
   are anything but a cold iceberg. If you've chosen
   romaine lettuce, you've got long leaves. Each has a bit of
   a spine. You may have to "crack it" a bit to stay flat.
   Remind yourself that you are flexible and capable of
   adjusting as needed.

6. Place one slice of onion on your sandwich. Onions often
   make us cry, and tears are a way of cleansing and
   letting go. Whether or not you actually cry or just think
   about a time you've cried, sit with the metaphor of
   letting go—of whatever you need to, but certainly of
   self-loathing and bitterness.

7. We continue with the letting-go metaphor by recognizing that there is a time to end a process, and we cover
   that up with "the meat of the matter." Yes, you should
   also "meat" yourself honestly. Meat can be tender and
   tough; likely, so can you. Name two things you are tender
   with and two where you are tough. Get to know and like
   the different textures of you. Meat is also rare or well
   done. First, name two things about yourself that are
   unique to you. Now, name two things you do well. We're
   focusing on accepting our perceived flaws as well as
   celebrating our strengths.

8. The final step is closure, always a great benefit in therapy and in life. As you place the bagel or bread on top,
   you are sealing in everything you learned about yourself and making a package, a gift to yourself. Press

down, pressing in the goodness of a new way of thinking, and remember the name of the session recipe, "Satisfied With Self Sandwich."

TO GO

Evaluate how this session worked for you. Here are some prompts for you to think about:

- Which steps were most impactful, and which metaphors might stick?
- As you go about your day, remember that change is possible. You can slice in a new presentation of yourself, set your intention and stick to it, let go of an old need to be perfect, be honest with yourself, and like yourself. Seal it all in as a gift from you to you.
- Take away a sense of ease at presenting yourself differently, and name two ways you might do this. Then take a mental picture of pressing down these actions into reality for muscle memory.

Refer back to this process as needed and especially if old triggers and thoughts return.

SCENIC DRIVE: Strut Your Stuff Saltimbocca

The need to present a perfect picture to the world is common for many of us and often learned in childhood. Comparing ourselves to others happens early and organically, in the classroom, on the sports fields, in the art room. It need not be unhealthy if perspective is a part of the recipe, meaning some of us excel in one arena, some in others.

However, maintaining this healthy outlook as we grow can prove challenging. The temptation to compare ourselves to others can take a truly destructive turn when we focus too much on what others think and not what makes us happy. We may see ourselves reflected in responses and reactions, a negative thought turns into a disparaging feeling, and suddenly it becomes a habit to care and adjust to the reactions of others. It's the beginning of acting falsely to please others. We may imagine that we need to be what others want us to be and feel ashamed of our true selves. We don a mask of competency when learning, surety when insecure, friendliness when tepid, and compliance while inwardly protesting, all in the service of getting along. We begin to lose the comfort of being ourselves, which can have emotional and even physical fallout. The masks become uncomfortable, too tight or too big to fill, and by absorbing too little of our own acceptance and too much of others perceived judgements, we hurt.

If you decide that what others think matters enormously, you will spend too much time trying to be what others want and less and less time discovering and being comfortable with who you are. Many clients come into therapy exclaiming, "I don't even know who I am or what I want anymore. I don't know how I got here!" There's good news: We can break this pattern. We can even love being "perfectly imperfect."

Start this session with guided imagery and a big cleansing breath. Literally. Right now. Then imagine yourself leaning over a pot of boiling water. Inhale all the steam, and imagine that steam is the negative nonsense you've inhaled for so long that makes you feel underachieving, faulty, or less than perfect. Turn away, and as you exhale, make a commitment to let that burning, churning, steam go and stop comparing yourselves to others. Do it twice if you find it helpful. And remember it the next time you default to fabricating or sugarcoating your situation. Remember, too, that many sweet dishes—like this chapter's first session, "It's Never All Smooth Smoothie" (page 125)—and most cookies and cakes do not need sugarcoating to be delicious, and neither do you.

Though I never want you to put your sweetness aside, we'll do just that for a moment for the next radical acceptance dish. Today's long, lazy recipe is for chicken saltimbocca. We'll call it "Strut Your Stuff Saltimbocca." This dish is filled with thinly sliced ingredients, but when we put them all together, we'll have a substantially thick dish. *Saltimbocca* literally means *jump in the mouth*, which is a perfect metaphor for taking a leap from envy and feeling diminished to flying your own fully fabulous flag.

Ingredients

4 chicken breasts	¼ cup white wine
Salt and pepper to taste	½ cup chicken broth
8 to 12 leaves fresh sage	3 tablespoons butter
4 slices prosciutto	Juice of 1 lemon
4 tablespoons olive oil	2 tablespoons flour

Session Instructions

1. Place each chicken breast between two pieces of plastic and pound to ¼-inch thickness. The pounding should remind you of all the voices in your head that

contributed to your need to appear perfect and how they made you so uncomfortable with your flaws.

2. Lightly salt and pepper the chicken. We are using salt for flavor but also to tenderize the meat. Think about how you can be more tender to yourself.

3. Layer a few slices of sage on each chicken breast. How great is it to have an ingredient called sage, as in sage advice or wisdom? As you press the sage into the chicken, press the idea into your head that you are enough, just the way you are.

4. To cement the idea of self-acceptance, now layer a slice of prosciutto on top of each chicken breast. We can think of the word *breast* here in terms of a breastplate, or the image you present to the world. Prosciutto takes a long time to "cure." Since we're using Italian meats, remind yourself that Rome wasn't built in a day, and emotions need time to cure too. It's a process and you've just begun.

5. Place the chicken in the fridge for a half hour to "come together" while you continue to let your thoughts of becoming self-accepting come together, sink in, and solidify.

6. Heat the oil in a pan over medium heat. As always, think about heat as a catalyst for change and the oil as malleable and fluid. Feelings are like that and do not have to stay fixed.

7. "Fit" the chicken into the pan, with the prosciutto side down, while thinking about being comfortable with a new fit of presenting yourself to the world. Take two to three minutes to let this sink in. Have a mindful moment by using your senses to "listen" to the noise of change and "smell" the deliciousness of the change.

8. Flip the chicken as you flip your idea of being perfect into one of self-love. Take two to three minutes and list

two to three imperfections that you can embrace with a thicker skin.

9. Remove the chicken to a plate and cover loosely. When we tent or cover loosely, we leave room for the heat to dissipate but also for the juices to remain. Think about being gentle in this way with yourself. No longer tightly wound, you can keep the good "juju" juices in and let the flaws and steam out.

10. Add the wine and broth to the pan and bring to a boil. Take note of the bubbles and the almost angry look and sound. This is what it's like when you are denigrating yourself. There is no gentle bubbling but rather a harsh and seething event. Lower the heat (and the judgment) and watch how the intensity lessens.

11. Add the butter and lemon together and acknowledge the softness and sharpness in all of us and the goodness of melting and being softer.

12. Sprinkle the flour into the pan to thicken and bind the sauce. Imagine yourself bolstered, your self-image solid, and all of the lessons of self-acceptance bound together.

13. Spoon and serve yourself bites as you "strut your stuff."

TO GO

Go from caring what others think to incorporating the sage wisdom that everyone has flaws and that's okay. Here is some more wisdom to bring into your reflections:

- Practice self-love by melting and binding together a new plan to acknowledge, celebrate, and become comfortable revealing your imperfections, which make you perfectly imperfect.

- Don't be chicken about making this change. Remember that most people are drawn to those who are imperfect because it lets them have flaws too.
- Think of all of your parts coming together and being flavorful despite sharpness (lemons) or mood changes (wine).

After-Dinner Mint

Remember, most traditional therapy sessions do not create breakthroughs in one session but rather after rapport has been established, comfort has been reached, and some of the thoughts and questions have had time to "marinate." This can happen days, weeks, and months later.

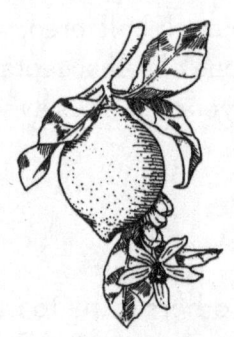

Chapter Nine

Session Four: Surviving Sadness

Pull up a chair, take a taste. Come join us. Life is so endlessly delicious.

—Ruth Reichl

Are you dealing with sadness or sorrow? This chapter is for you. Whether your sadness is related to a specific ongoing situation, an event, or an unexplained onset, you are not alone. As my mom used to say, "Into every life a little rain must fall."

Sadness can manifest in many ways. Some are subtle and physical. There, root causes need to be teased out, as in malaise, which is an overall sense of discomfort and feeling unwell and may be due to emotional or physical causes. Closely related to malaise is fatigue, which is an overwhelming and pervasive tiredness and lack of energy.

Once physical causes are ruled out, emotional conditions need to be explored. Even boredom can present as sadness, when lack of stimulation, often due to real-life transitions or events, occurs. Both anxiety and depression often present as sadness. Depression has been defined as "anger at self." It's generally accepted that many clients with depression may feel shame or inadequacy and turn those emotions inward, creating paralysis. But we must always remember that the brain is an organ, much like the lungs or kidneys, and imbalances exist that should and can be addressed to great improvement. Sometimes anxiety can be present in depression and vice versa. Sadness due to an event is thought to be transitory and, if dealt with, will resolve over time. The event might be a loss, an illness, or a life transition.

My practice in a women's wellness center exposed me to a wide range of clients adjusting to new roles. Some were new moms who loved their children but were overwhelmed and tired. They often looked enviously at single young women in the gym or at the supermarket, remembering freedom and flat stomachs. The latter concern may sound trite to some, but it was real for many. At the other end of the spectrum were clients whose children had left the nest. A whole stage of life had passed, and a sense of betrayal and loneliness ensued. Unlike the young moms, empty nesters, even when they were working outside the home, often asked, "What do I do now? Who needs me now?"

Life transitions such as new jobs or moves can create stress and/or loneliness. Prolonged routines can do the same, and malaise can be as paralyzing as extreme grief. Navigating life stages can be upending, and sadness is not unusual. In retiring adults, new roles need to be defined, and for the elderly there may be a sense that "the clock is ticking." For many, the idea of a "sunset of life" is anything but beautiful and feels more like a sunburn and rather scary. This group needs the sun to come *out*, not a sunset to emerge. In fact, anyone feeling gloomy or morose needs a sunrise.

It's important to distinguish between feelings of sadness and melancholy from a true diagnosis of clinical depression. In clinical depression, rumination, negative self-talk, and a prepondering dismal outlook for the future are prominent. Know there is no shame in any level of despair, whether it's prolonged or prominent. If you feel your sadness has crossed over into a debilitating state, where joy is absent, every day is filled with negative self-talk and excessive rumination, and the days seem endlessly difficult to manage, there *is* help for you. If you think you are suffering from depression and especially if you have thoughts of suicide, please reach out for help. Please see the Resources section at the end of the book for more (page 259).

> DEPRESSION HOTLINE USA: **Dial 988. Someone is there 24/7. Help exists, I promise.**

Let's proceed with our Fast Lane recipe, which I love to make at the "sunset" of a day but can also be made with yogurt if you need a morning boost.

> **As always, in each session remember to:**
> 1. Respect the space
> 2. Name the recipe (I've done it here for you)
> 3. Take stock of what you've brought to the table
> 4. Be present
> 5. Wash your hands before you begin

FAST LANE: Top It All Off Treat

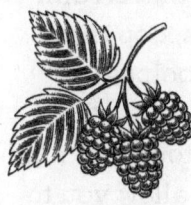

It's eight PM (or eight AM). The day is either ending or just beginning, and something must add a spark to your mood—and fast. You can work through that sense of heaviness or malaise with this easy and quick dish using ice cream (or yogurt) and toppings. I like to call it "Top It All Off Treat." By "top it all off," I mean finish the day (or start it) by letting all the negativity go and adding a bit of positive energy. I promise you it will make you smile and change your mood.

One more note: Have you heard about the rule of three? This is a principle suggesting that things that come in threes are inherently more satisfying and effective than those that come in any other number. We'll incorporate the rule of three during this session.

Ingredients

1 cup ice cream or frozen yogurt

At least three of the following toppings, or toppings of your choice:

Chocolate syrup

Chips, any kind (chocolate, white chocolate, peanut butter, etc.)

Mini marshmallows

Nuts

Multicolored sprinkles or something else colorful, like M&M's or tiny pieces of fruit, like kiwi or mango

Berries

Granola

Whipped cream

Session Instructions

1. As you scoop the ice cream or yogurt into a bowl, take a moment to enjoy its coolness, smoothness, and creaminess. Ask yourself what it would be like to scoop those three elements into your mind right now: coolness (about something you've been overly heated about?), smoothness (because of the bumps and detours life may be throwing at you?), creaminess (that will allow you to

regulate or soften your tone and talk to others and yourself?). You decide. This takes some practice. You can even lean down close to the bowl to feel the sensation of cold, or feel and notice the textures.

2. Imagine your thoughts, fears, and anxieties melting away as you see the ice cream or yogurt softening in the bowl.

3. Pick your first topping, which needs to be an item you can drop in: chips, marshmallows, nuts, berries, or granola. (Just don't use sprinkles, as that's going to be the next step.) Dropping in this topping will signify adding a drop of gratitude. For now, imagine your blessings, be they family, tangible goods or achievements, or inner strengths or qualities. We all have attributes and things we're proud of, so name three and say them out loud. Give yourself permission to refocus from any frustration or despondency to optimism and lightness.

4. The second topping is sprinkles. As you sprinkle, the operative word is color. Believe it or not, we can trick our minds in so many ways to generate new thought pathways. As you sprinkle, imagine your mind being overwhelmed with an infusion of color; imagine a fireworks display in your brain. It will spark a jolt of joy. Raise your head up to the sky to signify the light and bright colors spreading out into the universe but still staying within your brain.

5. Our third act is to "top it all off" with something to seal in the coolness, the color, and the consent to let the sun in. Pour syrup or squirt whipped cream, or if there's something else you'd like to add, this is a chance to be creative. Perhaps Magic Shell or peanut butter or melted caramel? There are so many ways to creatively seal in the session. Remember, creativity promotes happiness and improves overall mental health. So you be you!

6. Finally, take a mindful moment before your first spoonful to appreciate your efforts and the power of creating a simple but empowering dish. Truly pause and look at the bowl and feel proud. Let it boost your mood.

TO GO

If you began with profound sadness, I hope you were able to move a little bit toward feeling better. Here are some prompts for you as you reflect on your session:

- Were you able to incorporate the guided imagery?
- Did you take away a sense that you could change your thoughts?
- I give you permission to let the sun in by purposefully adding color, coolness, and creativity, which can work to change your mood and mindset.
- Remind yourself of blessings, sprinkling, and topping off—the rule of three in achieving happiness.
- Always take a mindful moment to admire and applaud; it's a game changer and makes for a sunny mood boost.
- Ask yourself honestly if this dish improved your mood. If so, commit to revisiting the steps.

EASY RIDER: Sheet Happens

A recipe that does double duty, just like cooking therapy, is a hit in my book and, of course, in my kitchen. This is a one-pan dish, meaning you can make your entire dinner in one sheet pan. I make this recipe or a version of it *a lot*. It will give you a fabulous dinner and also lift your spirits because it's easy, tasty, colorful, rich, and utilitarian. If you are someone who doesn't like to waste food, this recipe is for you. And hey, we all feel better when we aren't wasteful, right? But the main reason this dish is perfect for sparking a better mood is because it will make you smile and you'll never forget its name, I promise. I present to you: "Sheet Happens." Keep in mind that this dish will require a minimum of fifteen minutes' marinating time.

I use boneless, skinless thighs, but this recipe is great with any version of chicken, even breasts or a whole chicken cut up. Cooking time may vary, as you may need a bit longer for different parts—just make sure the internal temperature is 165°F.

I love to use color in my veggies for this dish, so I usually combine multicolor peppers, butternut squash cubes, onions, mushrooms, and snow peas. Sometimes sweet potatoes. Almost any vegetables work, so use whatever you have left over in the fridge or whatever suits your taste. If using sweet or regular potatoes, roast them for 10 minutes before adding the chicken to the sheet pan.

Ingredients

6–8 chicken thighs
½ cup soy sauce or tamari
½ cup maple syrup
½ cup Dijon (or other) mustard
4–6 cups raw vegetables, such as butternut squash, cubed; bell peppers, mushrooms, and onions, sliced; or snow peas
Olive oil or spray
Salt and pepper to taste

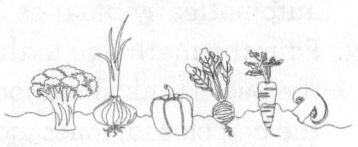

Session Instructions

1. Place the chicken thighs in a large Ziploc bag. This is a moment to think about taking your "troubles" and placing them somewhere other than your heart and mind. Therapists do this all the time with worry beads and boxes; they symbolically and tangibly remove worries by naming them, placing them on a bead, and then storing the worry bead in another container that is "disconnected" from being inside you. As you place each piece of chicken in the bag, name a feeling that's been bringing you down and attempt to remove it from inside you. This is a tangible visual help to "get the worry out" and put it somewhere where you can look at in a way that's more manageable.

2. Mix the soy sauce, syrup, and mustard together in a glass measuring cup. As you add each ingredient, think about how these three ingredients mirror life: The soy sauce is salty, the syrup is sweet, and the mustard is sharp. In life, we have moments of each. At some point, one flavor may outweigh the other, but for this recipe I'm purposely using equal amounts to suggest to you that you have the power to balance your emotions. Think especially about the sweet syrup balancing out the sharp and salty ingredients. How can you apply this to life? Pause for a mindful moment to think of a sweet blessing. When you focus mindfully on something positive, it can automatically balance out other troubles.

3. Pour the marinade in the bag with chicken and close the bag. Think about locking away those worries. With the bag closed, massage the marinade into the chicken pieces. This will tenderize the chicken. Tenderizing is

such a great word and metaphor, isn't it? You are changing the hardness of each piece and each worry. You are turning them into something softer and something that can more easily absorb flavor. Don't be too quick about the task. Quite simply, you are tenderizing yourself.

4. Zip up the bag and marinate it in the fridge. The longer the better, but even fifteen minutes will give you a delicious dish. If you have the time, marinate for at least an hour or even up to overnight. Either way, the chicken takes time to absorb the flavors, and you'll take some time to absorb different self-talk. You can sit with these suggestions for however long you'd like. They may take hold instantly or over weeks. Problems don't disappear at the same rate for everyone.

5. Collect the vegetables. Any will do; go for a balance of color and shape. Line a sheet pan with parchment paper and place all the vegetables on it. Here's an example of what to use:

- Butternut squash, in small cubes no bigger than ½ inch. Think about your concerns being like these cubes, broken down into manageable parts instead of one big overwhelming mess. And of course, squash the big ones if you can.

- Three colors of bell peppers, thinly sliced. They can be red, yellow, orange, or green; sliced, whole, or the mini ones in a bag. If you are slicing your own, think about "slices of life" and how many days make up a life. Not every day will be sad; some will be colorful like these peppers. If using the packaged peppers, grab a few of them by the short stalk for a moment and think about how you are in control (you might even swing them around a bit to make the point) and how you can decide what to place in your life. It might refer to people, hobbies, or goals. We are going for positive, colorful, sunny choices.

- Mushrooms. Mushrooms are full of water and will change dramatically in consistency when roasted. In this dish, they provide a fantastic metaphor for letting go. Let the heaviness drain as you think about how these mushrooms will go from hard and firm to soft and malleable, losing their water but not their substance. These will cook a lot faster than the other ingredients and be a little more done, but I don't mind. If we can be a little more "done" with whatever problems we're dealing with, that's ideal.

- Onions. There's no secret sauce to why we're using this ingredient. Emotions must come out, and I'd love it if you allow yourself to cry a little while slicing or chopping these. If you really want a good cry, I find that red onions are sharper. Long ago I heard an expression that if you don't share your feelings verbally, then eventually they will "come out the neck." Essentially this means that it's unhealthy to keep feelings, and especially secrets, inside. If you don't talk about them, they can show up as physical pain, mental health issues, or impulsive words or actions. Cry it out when making this dish. If possible, identify one or two actual reasons that make you cry. When you're done, be done. Wipe your eyes, cool them with water, have a mindful moment to feel what it's like to let go, and move on.

- Snow pea pods. I love snow pea pods in this recipe because they are simply bursting with goodness. Sign me up for that! And what's inside? Big beautiful green seeds. These seeds are so reflective of possibility and change, both in texture and color, and they are so full inside the pod it's like they're just bursting to get out. If nothing else, take away the image of these snow pea pods as nature's creation of growth and life, and try to think about bursting into your own life instead of coasting along.

6. Mix all the vegetables together on the parchment-lined sheet pan, spread them out and spray or drizzle them with olive oil, then add salt and pepper. Whether you are spraying or drizzling the oil, it will add softness and help the vegetables release their juices. Try to release the pain and/or stagnation that's bringing you down and remind yourself of your flavors (natural gifts and abilities). The salt and pepper are sprinklings of even more flavors (ideas of creating joy). Mix it all in.

7. Preheat the oven to 425 degrees. This dish takes a high level of heat, which might reflect the way you've been feeling your intense emotions. As always, turning on the oven to any temperature reminds us that heat is a catalyst for change and that you've made an effort to change. Remember, too, that just as emotions change, stages in life always change, and what you're feeling right now will not be what you'll be feeling in a day, a month, or a year from now. Just like with this oven, we will eventually press OFF and the heat will dissipate.

8. Remove the chicken pieces from the bag, layer them on top of the veggies, and discard the marinade. Think about how many layers there are in a day, in the course of a life, and of course, in you. Highlight any negativity you may have been able to discard during this session. You may choose to let the chicken sit for a few minutes to lose the chill. This will be an additional opportunity

for you to imagine your emotions warming up and filling you with self-love rather than sadness.

9. Place the sheet pan in the oven and cook for thirty minutes or until the chicken is browned, its internal temperature is 165, and the veggies are soft and tender. Remove and observe. The vegetables are flavorful and they have absorbed the chicken juices and marinade. The chicken is golden and tender. I'll guess that your "Sheet Happens" recipe looks amazing.

10. As you let the chicken rest for five to ten minutes, it's a chance for you to rest, in more ways than one. First, you can rest from your physical efforts. Wipe your brow, grab a favorite drink, and relax. Next, and more important, think about giving the fuel of negativity and debilitating thoughts a rest. Perhaps this recipe can serve as a visual and reminder every time your mind goes down a path of sadness or despair. Then, when the juices of the chicken are sealed inside, think about sealing in this new way of loving yourself.

11. In this Easy Rider session, you were asked to "prepare" to face some difficult subjects. Take a moment to applaud your efforts and the result. You did it! I hope you have absorbed at least a bit of "happy juice" going forward and are feeling sunnier than at the start.

TO GO

Remember that "sheet happens" but you have the tools to overcome it when it does. Here is some advice for you as you reflect on this session:

- Be tender with yourself.
- Chop your problems into manageable parts.

- Choose to absorb all the juices in life but always aim for balance and remember that life cooks quickly and "slices" of it change.
- Have you been feeling raw? If so, try to internalize the visual of heating for change and cooking up a more palatable state as well as eventually turning the heat of the moment down.
- It's important to remind yourself of your individual and beautiful colors and flavors.
- You will hear me say often that we ruminate, sometimes endlessly, over perceived failures but take so little time to let the successes live and seep into our thoughts. It's certainly a most unequal balance and a habit we should work to change. Start with self-talk: *I'm enough.* Let that create a feeling: *I feel capable and lovable.* Move to a behavior: *I'll call that new friend* or *I'll try that gym.*

SCENIC DRIVE: Perspective Popovers

Remember Sophie, the teenage girl who thought everyone had it more together than she did? That kind of skewed view can lead to so many negative emotions. Social media is a pet peeve of mine; many of us, teens or not, can be leveled by insecurity and sadness from watching the rose-colored and doctored photos of others.

Feeling good about ourselves and our lives shouldn't have to be an exercise in extreme intervention, so a little perspective helps. Perspective can be a sword or a gift. You have the ability to decide how to frame events and how you feel about them. One of the very first cooking therapy sessions I ever created is your Scenic Drive. It's called

"Perspective Popovers" and packs a big punch of attitude adjustment by showing you just how much your perspective can be faulty, and also how it can be altered to be your friend.

You'll need a six-cup popover or muffin pan for this recipe.

Ingredients

1¼ cup flour
¼ teaspoon salt
3 large eggs
1¼ cup milk

2 tablespoons unsalted butter, cut into six even pieces
1 tablespoon unsalted butter, melted

Session Instructions

1. Spray your pan with nonstick spray and think about unsticking your current view or emotion about something that's bothering you. Think about letting go of old ideas you've been stuck to, especially negative feelings or worries.

2. Preheat the oven to 400 degrees, and as always, think about heat as a catalyst for change. When we're stuck in a sad state, it's hard to change. Stare at the oven for a moment. It takes time to "heat up" and reach the optimum temperature. The same is true for you to truly try on a new perspective. It may go slowly, but stay with it. As you stare at the oven heating up and changing temperature, you can too.

3. Measure the flour and put it into a bowl. Think about taking measure of all that's good in your life. Name three to four blessings out loud. For example, you might say, "I have great kids," "I have great parents," or "I have great friends"; "I have a stable job"; "I have

people who are kind to me and who I'm kind to"; or "I'm creative," "I'm a problem solver," or "I'm excellent at _____" (you fill in the blank). After this, would you be able to clap for yourself with powdery hands? It's a silly but wonderful way to affirm blessings and joy and to be childish in a good way.

4. Add the salt and allow yourself to acknowledge a part of your life that may not be working. Tell yourself that in time you'll be able to change this and address whatever obstacle is blocking your progress or standing in your way.

5. Crack the eggs and think about new life and "birthing" new ideas. Things will get better. Life is not stagnant, and adding eggs is an opportunity to tangibly state to yourself that change happens. If a few pieces of eggshell get in, no problem. Use it as an additional metaphor for healing as you take them out. (And revisit my trick for removing eggshells from page 83.)

6. Add the milk, and using an electric mixer, blend all the ingredients into a smooth and cool mixture. First, focus on the noise. This is how we all get at times in our heads. I call it "brain on puree"; it's that worry loop or negative self-talk. Instead, look at the new mixture. This is exactly how you might think of yourself going forward, as someone who can be newly blended, cool, and content, smoothly handling any emotional bumps or triggers or worries or fears.

7. Place the pan in the oven for two minutes to warm, and while waiting, practice positive self-talk, like "I've had enough of feeling sad, and I deserve to feel better" and "I'm fully capable of change."

8. Remove the pan from the oven. Add a piece of butter to each of the six popover cups and put the pan back in

the oven just for a minute to melt the butter. Think about all the pieces of you softening and melting into a calm and happy state. Set a timer for one minute. Close your eyes and have a mindful full minute of a breathing session. First, as slowly as you can, breathe in for a count of eight. Then, just as slowly, breathe out for the same eight counts. You should be able to do this three to four times in one minute. You will feel your body and mind becoming peaceful. Tie that feeling to a visualization of yourself at peace. What does that feel like?

9. Remove the pan from the oven, and fill each cup halfway with batter. Imagine filling yourself up with all the steps prior: adding positive self-talk, integrating coolness and smoothness, feeling warm and wonderful. Bake for twenty minutes. While the popovers are baking, say ten times out loud, "It will be okay."

10. After twenty minutes, turn the oven temperature down to 300 degrees and continue baking for another twenty minutes. Remind yourself that you are completely capable of turning down the noise in your mind and negative feelings that "pop up." In addition, cement the new idea that not only can you turn down negative feelings, but you can also "turn up" a feeling of joy just as easily as turning up the dial on the oven.

11. Finally, remove the popovers and admire your work. The popovers should look like fluffy mushrooms with a flaky, large top. Don't they look great? Enjoy the mastery. Take a full five minutes to look at the popovers, and during that time tell yourself that you are amazing. It might seem like a long time to compliment yourself, but remember how easy it is to ruminate about sadness or perceived failures. So take the time and enjoy your creation. Also the popovers. ☺

12. Cut into one of the popovers. What do you see? Beautiful pastry work (that's you), but also, they are quite airy. The next time you are thinking that someone else is happier, remember, they might just look that way on the outside, while inside, that may not be the case at all. Now that's a visual that has "perspective" legs!

TO GO

Here are some prompts for you to consider as you think about your session:

- Do you think you can attempt to "cook up" a different perspective? Going forward, name one or two ways you'll do this.
- Were you able to integrate the idea of turning down the heat after a while and also turning up joy? Name a situation where you might.
- Try to remember to pause if feel your perspective becoming skewed and creating sadness or worry.

Refer back to this recipe session as needed.

After-Dinner Mint

Remember, most traditional therapy sessions do not create breakthroughs in one session but rather after rapport has been established, comfort has been reached, and some of the thoughts and questions have had time to "marinate." This can happen days, weeks, and months later.

Chapter Ten

Session Five: The Courage To Change

It's okay to play with your food.

—Emeril Lagasse

In fencing, and especially in boxing, pivoting means "feinting" left or right to avoid the punches. It can mean the difference between taking a blow to the jaw or avoiding the punch. This is such a powerful prescription for all of us for so many moments in life. Rather than being rigid and hoping to hold on to the smooth straightaways, life is so much more about learning to be flexible and navigate the bumps and detours, which I promise will come.

Years ago, I had a needlepoint pillow that said *Bloom Where You're Planted*. I loved that pillow and that mantra, and for a long time I subscribed to that saying because it meant I should make the best of things. However, the older I got and the more clients I saw, the more I realized that too many people were stuck in negative communication loops, emotional battlefields, repeated martyrdom, rigid mindsets, and ineffective patterns as well as actual jobs or relationships. Eventually, I turned the pillow over and adopted a new saying: *Bloom Where You're Planted. Or Move.* I don't think they cancel each other out but instead suggest two different plans for two different moments.

There is a time to *move*. Together we can explore the components that lead up to making a move, but only you can decide if the time is right. Not everyone who explores a change makes one. There is benefit in evaluating. For some, the situation is clear, and they decide to stay where they are, and yet for others, the old saying applies: "Something's gotta give."

Think of a teapot on the stove. The whistle goes off and we run to shut the noise. But we don't often think about the science of what's going on inside the teapot. The water heats, it bubbles and boils, and there is so much steam that it needs to be released, and the spout opens from the pressure and the steam literally blows its top with a resounding noise.

If you've been stuck in a pressured situation and the steam has nowhere to go, this chapter, primarily about external pressures, is for you. We discussed many internal pressures in Chapter 5, session one, "Creating Calm." These are often self-imposed by perfectionism, worry, or misguided thoughts and create anxiety or stress. External pressures, however, are those assigned to outside situations such as a job or relationship or lifestyle. Parsing through is the work we'll do in session five. Any situation that makes you feel degraded or devalued or disgruntled is a situation that needs to change.

This chapter is also about feeling stuck from outside choices you may have made to survive, or for someone else, or by mistake, or because you were young, and now are creating all sorts of negative emotions and maybe even actions. Here we'll talk about tangible situations and try to evaluate and crystallize whether it's time to make a change.

The key phrase is *crystalizing thoughts*. Think of the teapot. We'll look at those inner and increasingly active bubbles and growing heat and try to determine how to bring them down to a manageable and clear simmer of choices and options. This chapter is about conversation, not action.

Life has a way of *living us* at times, rather than the other way around. My kids tell their little girls, ages two and five, "You be you!" But detours happen as we grow older, and sometimes even before we fully know who we are or what we want, we wonder what's happened and why we are no longer doing "us being us."

If you're finding it difficult to bloom, then the recipes to come will help. By the end of this chapter, you'll be able to view your situation calmly and with a clear lens so you can proceed.

As always, in each session remember to:

1. Respect the space
2. Name the recipe (I've done it here for you)
3. Take stock of what you've brought to the table
4. Be present
5. Wash your hands before you begin

FAST LANE: Priority Pasta

I created this recipe for a corporate cooking therapy session and was initially told that the employees wanted to explore the idea of work/life balance. Prior to the actual date of the presentation, I received several calls from two of the liaisons at the company, and I sensed that many in the group might be feeling undervalued rather than under-balanced. Knowing that employees are often fearful about leaving or staying at a company, as each option comes with its own risk, I pivoted in my presentation plan and aimed it at priorities at work rather than creating a work/home balance. It was a slight change but opened a discussion about work practices that might otherwise have gone unaddressed.

This recipe will help you evaluate priorities and make an informed choice. That's why I call it "Priority Pasta." It reminds me of a quote from the book "Harold and the Purple Crayon" by Crockett Johnson (1955): "Harold wanted to go into the forest, but he didn't want to get lost in the woods, so he built a forest with just one tree." That quote and the ingredients in this dish may make you laugh, but they do speak to making informed choices, and also, I've always said that I could do cooking therapy with just one ingredient.

Ingredients

1 packaged macaroni and cheese cup, such as Kraft

Session Instructions

1. Shake the cup. It makes a lot of noise. Do you feel like you are experiencing jumbles of frustrations or questions or concerns? Carly Simon wrote about reducing the noise in our head. Decide right now to do the same. With a bunch of noise, we can't explore the one or two things that are changeable.
2. Peel off the top and think about peeling back the cover on what's underneath. Remove the cheese packet and set it aside. Look at the macaroni. It's hard and raw. Notice how it isn't soft or flexible. Decide if this is the way you feel right now. If so, we're going to do our best to change that.

3. Add water to the fill line. Think of one or two things that do fill you up or might fill you up and could soften this hard "inside" of your cup. It could be at work, at home, or generally in your life. Say it out loud or to yourself: "This fills me up." If you can't come up with anything, that's equally telling. If that's the case, think of two things you'd like to add to your cup that would fill you up.

4. Place the cup in the microwave and cook according to the directions on the package. As always, heat is the ultimate catalyst for change, converting so many dishes from one state to another. Think about the same for you while you wait. Consider the possibilities of changing what's not working. Don't simply name feelings but name actual elements that could change.

5. Remove from the microwave and add the cheese packet, thinking even more about adding and sprinkling even small ways you could change your situation for the better. If you're stuck, no clearer on options than when you began, don't worry. You've already begun to con-template, and crystallized ideas may come in days or weeks ahead. Stir gently, being kind to yourself about this. If you have uncovered an idea or two, notice as you stir that the macaroni is now soft and malleable, as you may be too.

6. Once the mac and cheese has "come together," it's superhot, and I like to pop an ice cube in to bring down the heat and make the dish eatable. A dish or a situation that is too hot will burn you. But if you cool it down, you'll be able to gobble up the new ideas. Continue stirring until the ice cube melts, and decide not only when the cup is ready but if/when you might be ready to change or soften your situation.

TO GO

"Priority Pasta" is a call to contemplation. You can take your feelings and crystallize them so you can think and act clearly. You may make a change, the way the macaroni does, but the ice cube at the end also gives you the freedom to simply chill on the idea. Here are some more prompts for you to ponder:

- Try to identify two quiet or internal needs you'd like to address, instead of just feeling a free-floating emotion, like a great ball of noise. If you can, say them aloud to cement.
- Ask yourself, what fills you? This is an important piece in decision-making.
- Which step in this recipe was the most helpful to you?
- If you began the recipe feeling disjointed, indecisive, or confused, have you clarified any options? If so, remember, no need to become anxious when choices are hard; simply soften by pausing and filling yourself with notions of what matters to you, then chill on it.

EASY RIDER: Frittata Transformata

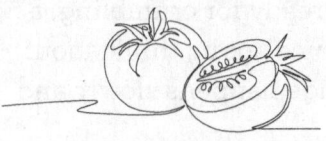

If you're like me, breakfast for dinner is on the menu any day of the week. I've chosen this recipe especially for this chapter on contemplating a change, because it has six eggs. By now you know that I think eggs are a huge symbol of birth and coming alive and certainly producing new ideas. Also, I think they're a reminder, six times, that you are a "good egg" just the way you are. And even though it's an uncomplicated recipe, it does have "mix-ins." Isn't that perfect for deliberating, perhaps with a pros-and-cons list? We'll have fun and we'll be purposeful, especially as we watch this recipe "change" from loose to solid. I call it "Frittata Transformata." You will need an oven safe pan or a two-quart baking dish for this recipe.

Ingredients

6 slices precooked bacon
6 extra-large eggs
¾ cup milk of your choice
2 tablespoons butter, melted
Salt, pepper, and garlic
    powder to taste

½ cup chopped scallions
½ cup cherry tomatoes
1¼ cup shredded cheese of
    your choice

Session Instructions

1. Preheat your oven to 350 degrees. Let's talk about the number 350, which is *almost* 360. "Doing a 360" means you're going to make a complete turnaround, 360 degrees, and it's the perfect way to think about the start of "transforming."
2. Lay the precooked bacon on a pan and place it in the oven. You are getting the bacon ready for crumbling, a change from its original state. Once again, think about readiness and preparation. Change happens slowly and in stages.
3. While the bacon is heating up, crack each of the six eggs into a bowl. Every time you crack an egg, name one thing you'd like to change. Simply name each thing. Although the eggs are extra large, your "change items" might be small, such as "laugh more" or "drink more

water." When you make even small changes, they have a way of exponentially giving you power you didn't know you had.

4. Add the milk and melted butter to the bowl. How does it change the eggs? Does the mixture look different, perhaps looser or a different color? Are there swirls? It's not quite clear yet what this dish will be; it hasn't come together yet. That's exactly what happens when you make a change. Living with uncertainty may be new, but it's a part of life. Take a mindful moment to embrace the feeling and infuse yourself with strength to manage it.

5. Are you ready for a great visual and tangible task? Add the salt, pepper, and garlic to *your* liking, and then whisk everything together in the bowl. As you do so, think about the power in your hands. Now everything is coming together, even though it takes some work on your part.

6. Remove the bacon from the oven and set it aside with the other ingredients. "Setting aside" is a metaphor. Think about what you've put "on the back burner" that's kept you from a more fulfilling life. Take a mindful moment for this.

7. Pour the mixture into the pan or baking dish. This is your life now, your base. We're going to add items, beginning with the bacon. Crumble it and sprinkle it on top of the egg mixture. Do not think of negative crumbling. Instead, think of what you can do right now to add to your life. Bacon is salty and tangy. It's flavorful. We all need flavor, not just a base. Do this with each of the next ingredients, from scallions to tomatoes, imagining the base of your frittata becoming colorful and interesting.

8. Finally, cover the entire pan or dish with the shredded cheese. Having "the cheese" is often a metaphor for

getting everything you want in life. There was even a successful self-help book called *Who Moved my Cheese?* about the ever-changing "'maze" of life and navigating change. What about "the big cheese"? It's a bit narcissistic, but why not be the big cheese, be in charge of your own life, as if it's a company? I knew an executive who had a business card, and under his name it said "Le Grand Fromage." That's French for *the big cheese.* Clearly he had success and a sense of humor. Look at your covered dish and imagine the change you'd like to make to "add the cheese."

9. Place in the preheated oven for approximately thirty minutes or until the center is no longer visibly wobbly or jiggly, the edges are golden brown, and if you gently shake the pan, the egg mixture appears set with only a slight movement in the middle. How about you? Are you feeling a bit more set and less wobbly? As you cut a slice of your "Frittata Transformata," I hope you will feel a bit "transformated" and filled with "egg-celent" ideas and thoughts about change and how it fits into your life. Sorry, that was "cheesy," but I couldn't resist.

TO GO

Change looks swirly and loose at the beginning but comes together eventually. You have the power to "whisk" smoothness into your life. Here are some prompts for you as you process this session:

- Sprinkling is a metaphor for crystallizing your thoughts and adding change elements.

- You've got all the ingredients, the base, the flavorful fillings, and the top. Do not accept crumbs; being the "big cheese" in your own life is doable.
- Ask yourself if this frittata did in fact create a "transformata" and if you are more ready to contemplate or enact helpful changes. If so, affirm the process by congratulating yourself on quite a masterful dish (I mean you).

Return to the session as needed to remind yourself that change is possible.

SCENIC DRIVE: Unset in Your Ways Stromboli

Years ago, I quit smoking. It wasn't easy. I had tried many ways to quit, but eventually it was a CBT-based program called Smokenders that did the trick. In the program, I learned that my firm thoughts were incorrect. For instance, I called some of the cigarettes my especially "good" cigarettes. These were the ones that came after a meal or coffee, while driving, or when I was on the phone. I learned instead that the minute I put one cigarette out, my body went into withdrawal, and so any cigarette I had after that wasn't a "good" one but simply a relief from the pain. A relief from the pain of withdrawal. Can you say *aha* moment?

The minute I thought about it differently, I saw the cigarettes differently. Even more, the instructor likened each cigarette to an aspirin, a common relief from pain, and he asked, "Would you ever take an aspirin and say, 'Man, that was some good aspirin'?" Funny thought, but instantly powerful. I would never see another cigarette as "good" again.

There were other parts of the program that asked you to examine the benefits of your habit. One was cost. What was it costing you—financially, healthwise, timewise, and in terms of internal self-image—to smoke?

Imagine the cost benefit of continuing a habit, behavior, or lifestyle that doesn't serve you well versus making a change. One more thought before we begin: The musical group Blessid Union of Souls suggested in one of their songs that when you face the things that scare you, that's where self-discovery is revealed. Think about that as we prepare "Unset in Your Ways Stromboli."

Ingredients

Flour for dusting
1 pound package frozen pizza dough (often found in the bakery section), brought to room temperature
1 package thin-sliced salami
1 package sliced provolone cheese

1 package prosciutto
½ cup shredded mozzarella cheese, skim okay
Garlic powder
Oregano
1 egg
1 tablespoon water

Session Instructions

1. Flour a clean work surface. Just as we prepare for the session by checking in with what we've brought to the table and you are getting ready to receive insight and awareness, the flour is getting ready to receive the dough. Take a breath to internalize readiness.
2. The dough is more workable at room temperature (what isn't?). If you need to wait a bit, prepare the other ingredients by removing them from their packages.
3. Preheat the oven to 425 degrees. Waiting and heating are two metaphors for determining. Waiting can

be thought of as the first step in the change cycle, precontemplation, while heating has a bit more action, moving you right into the next step, contemplation.

4. Stretch and knead the dough just a bit. This will make it easier to roll out. Try to just stretch it enough to make it easier to roll but not tear. Think about how you stretch yourself in so many directions and whether you do so without tearing. Take a moment to feel the raw dough. Ask yourself *Where do I feel raw and what do I knead/need?* Really think about an answer.

5. With a rolling pin, roll out the dough to a rectangle, approximately 12 × 16. Add more flour to the surface and rolling pin as needed so the dough doesn't stick. Imagine a choice or change you've been contemplating. Adding more flour represents adding ideas to help you plan more smoothly and to make that plan stick together. Don't just think about the change, think about the plan you will enact. Rolling out the dough takes a little work. This part of the plan requires the same. If there wasn't some conflict or adjustment, the change wouldn't be difficult to make.

6. Time to layer, one of my favorite cooking therapy steps! Place the salami on the dough, slightly overlapping, leaving about an inch of room all around. This is what I call your escape route! The inch of dough is so the ingredients don't fall out once rolled. Think about that idea of "being contained." At any point in deciding to make a change, you can "roll back" the idea and let the choice itself change. You can escape your own plan. But if you are becoming resolved, then the more you layer your decisions and keep them an inch in, the more they will be contained.

7. Continue layering with the provolone and prosciutto, repeating your options and thinking about the layers of you that have contributed or may be engaged by making this change. Have you grown in ways that allow you to make this change? More strength? Confidence? Resolve? Name these attributes out loud. It's okay if you feel as if you're still trying to employ them or even if you feel that where you are right now is not ready. Sometimes just by naming what we want, we get closer to having it.

8. Sprinkle the shredded mozzarella over the layers. Try to name concrete steps required for your change. Think about how the cheese will melt and seal in all the steps and also the layers and the parts of you that are connected. Sprinkle in oregano and garlic to taste, and sprinkle in anything you're still not sure about such as risks, timelines, effort, and cost. If you're deliberating about a more internal change such as confidence, calm, open-mindedness, or patience, the cost may be less consequential but still a challenge.

9. Time to roll with it. Not only are we rolling up all the thoughts, work, options, considerations, and decisions we may have made, but take a breath now and tell yourself that you are ready to roll, in more ways than one. As you roll the dough, starting from the long side, keep pinching in the ends so the ingredients don't fall out, as we discussed in step four. Remind yourself that you are a unique combination of many layers and ingredients, and so is the decision to make any transform. Keeping all those steps inside the stromboli is an affirmation that you are also "together."

10. Once rolled, place the stromboli seam side down on a cookie sheet lined with parchment paper or nonstick

aluminum foil. Whisk the egg (always a metaphor for whipping up new ideas) and the water with a fork and brush the mixture over the top and sides of the stromboli. You are sealing in not only your ideas but the work you did. This is incredible mastery. Look at your creation. Pause to admire for a solid minute.

11. Now sprinkle a bit more oregano and garlic on top and place on the bottom rack of the oven. This is important. The stromboli does better with room to rise. We all do better with room to rise. After all of the steps, ask yourself if the change you're contemplating will give you more or less room to rise. This will help you discover if it's time to become "unset" in the aspect of yourself you want to change, or not.

12. Bake the stromboli for approximately twenty-five minutes or until the top is browned. Remove from the oven and let it rest for at least ten minutes before slicing. This is so important. Take these ten minutes to reflect on your work and your achievement once again.

13. When you slice the stromboli, visualize all the layers of you and the work you've done in contemplating change. Whether you stay "set" or "unset" is up to you; but whatever you decide, great job.

TO GO

Here are some reminders as you contemplate change:

- Change requires both patience and a ramp-up or heating to be ready. You can weigh your options, layer your choices and strengths, and either let go of your ideas or contain them and keep going.

- It may be surprising to think of change as hard work. Always roll with it, too, and stretch yourself.
- Remember that human beings are capable of taking on different shapes, and at the same time it's okay to be "kneady."
- Give yourself a chance to decide if you have room to rise, but remember that all of us can rise if we add or subtract the right ingredients.
- Sprinkle in steps to take or attributes of yourself that either contribute or detract from your ability to change. Then remain "set" or "unset" in your ways, and don't let the lessons you've learned leak out.

After-Dinner Mint

Remember, most traditional therapy sessions do not create breakthroughs in one session but rather after rapport has been established, comfort has been reached, and some of the thoughts and questions have had time to "marinate." This can happen days, weeks, and months later.

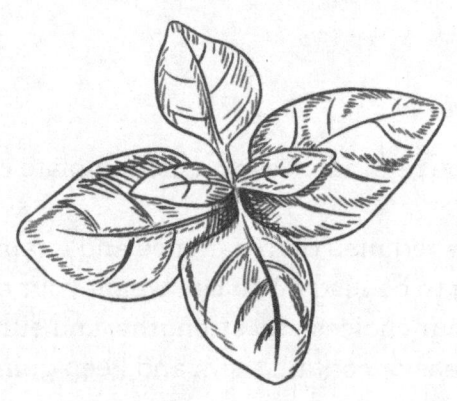

Chapter Eleven

Session Six: How to Hear and Be Heard

You learn a lot about someone when you share a meal together.

—Anthony Bourdain

What we tell ourselves—our self-talk—significantly determines how we feel and what we do. The secret sauce is achieved when we remove the ingredients that don't taste right and add in the flavors that do. Learning to improve all dialogue requires adaptation, flexibility, and a willingness to experiment, similar to the way a chef cooks. But there's power in knowing that you already have the tools to do it. In this chapter we'll examine all types of discourse, the kind that's in our head and the kind we use with others.

The way we communicate is often ingrained, learned in our families of origin, and cemented, even if it's faulty. Everyone wants to be able to convey what they mean, need, or want, but often emotions or style gets in the way. Adding cooking therapy to an overall excavation of these patterns can create a visual and tangible tool.

For this reason, let's look at communication styles in terms of the ingredients in your "pantry." Everyone has canned goods, but have yours expired? Meaning are you repeating the same phrases, words, or admonitions over and over again and still feeling unheard or ineffective? Your phrases may be "past their best used by" date, like items that have been hiding way in the back forever. These are unusable and no one can eat them, aka take them in. These cans might even have bulging tops, ready to blow. They are toxic in your pantry and toxic for your relationships. When we identify and replace old goods with fresher ones, we experience delight. If we swap out those old beans with couscous, for example, everyone is pleasantly surprised, but more, they can hear you. And this is ultimately the goal of any therapy: understand what's not working, then change a pattern for more success.

Before we dive into the recipes, let's do a simple activity called the miracle question, which is often used by therapists to help their clients crystallize goals and feelings. It's a simple imagination technique, a set of questions that helps clients to imagine a problem being solved or removed and can motivate them toward their own solutions.

The Miracle Question Activity

1. Sit in a comfortable chair in a dark and quiet room with your feet on the ground.
2. Place your hands in your lap and close your eyes.
3. Take a cleansing breath.
4. Now pretend that during the night, while you were sleeping, a wonderful miracle happened. When you woke up in the morning, how would you know? What would you see and feel? What would be different?
5. Open your eyes and take a few moments to think about your answers to the questions. What was the miracle?

Although many clients express that they'd have the job of their dreams, a relative's illness eradicated, a dream house, or an improved partnership, I've also noticed when using the miracle question that many clients talk about a relative who's passed or a relationship that's broken. They say things like "John would still be here beside me" or "Rachel and I would be speaking again" or "Jeremy and the kids wouldn't have moved to California and would still be living around the corner." Did that happen for you? I've learned that so much of what matters to us is about *who* is in our life, *how* they are in our life, and *what* we can do to keep those connections strong and positive.

While we can't resurrect loved ones, we *can* use processes and metaphors to move us toward the goal of positive communication in all our relationships, including the relationship we have with ourselves. For this reason, remember your goals when talking to someone. Is it just to get something off your chest or to get something accomplished? Is it to hear yourself state your point of view or to hear another's? Many people get frustrated and snap and ruin relationships. And yet, if you ask them what their goal was prior to snapping, they will often say it was to get their point across in order to have a better relationship. This is so sad. Reworking these faulty wires can result in so much happiness. You know you can't change other people, but you can certainly learn to reality-check your own style and decide if you'd like to change. Maybe you will, maybe you won't. That part is up to you.

Sometimes, when we're in cooking therapy, we have to "cut off the hard parts" of an ingredient, such as celery or kale. Other times we need to "soften" an item, such as butter for baking, vegetables for a soup, or even ice cream. Certain meats, such as beef or chicken, will cook much better when they sit out for a half hour and "lose their cold a bit." Examining our communication styles may mean looking at all those metaphors. Is our style "hard" and inflexible and, consequently, "hard to hear"? Do we need to soften finite language or our tone in expressing our needs? Is there a time to simply take our thoughts from icy to room temperature before they become words? We will examine all of these in the cooking therapy sessions below.

Additionally, these concepts must be applied to communication between you and you, not just between you and others. I love that phrase "between you and you." So often we forget that the majority of the time what we tell ourselves determines our mood, our manner of behaving, and our feelings of self-worth. Believe it or not, this even has an effect on how we communicate with others. Self-doubt, or worse, self-loathing, can have a ripple effect. When we're operating from a perch of negative self-worth, it can cause us to speak in ways we don't intend, from sharply to meekly. Be gentle with yourself. Speak lovingly to yourself. Remind yourself often of your strengths and successes. This will help you in numerous ways, including how you get your point across and achieve your goals.

In Chapter 10 I told you about an experience I had quitting smoking, where I had to think about cigarettes in a different way; not as "good" and delicious but as "aspirins" simply curing pain. But additionally, in order to deal with the urges that comes with changing a habit, I had to change my self-talk. In the past, when I had felt the urge for a cigarette, I'd say, "I'm feeling that I want a cigarette." My new thought was different. I'd say, "Ah, I recognize this feeling. In the past, this is when I'd have a cigarette, but now I do something else." Very subtle but powerful. And this is exactly how we change a communication style internally and externally. We get the urge to repeat a pattern, but instead we stop, recognize that the pattern has been ineffective, and try on a new one. Ultimately, it's not a full pantry makeover but a swapping out of some old ingredients, and it does the trick.

As always, in each session, remember to:

1. Respect the space
2. Name the recipe (I've done it here for you)
3. Take stock of what you've brought to the table
4. Be present
5. Wash your hands before you begin

FAST LANE: Adjustment Avocado Toast

Have you had the experience of trying to get your point across without being heard? If you're only focused on your own point of view rather than listening to what another person is saying, things are not likely to change, and compromise will be elusive.

Here is an example of communication gone awry between a mother and daughter. Seventeen-year-old Heather and her mom are constantly at odds. The mom is distraught. While they once had a close relationship, now that Heather has her driver's license, her mother feels things have changed. Heather has very different ideas about rules than her mom does, specifically in terms of her curfew. Her mother wants Heather home at ten PM, and Heather says, "She's crazy." It usually ends with Heather running into her room and slamming the door while her mom shouts, "I'm still in charge."

The problem here is less about curfew and more about a miscommunication. Heather's mom is saying *I'm struggling with this new change, I love you so much, and I'm terrified that something bad will happen to you.* Heather is hearing *Mom treats me like a baby and wants to make me a prisoner because she doesn't trust me or think I'm capable.* Without an intervention, this miscommunication can play out endlessly. Ultimately, Heather's mom will set and enforce her rules, and Heather may comply or disobey, but whatever happens, both will feel frustrated and the relationship may become further strained. Moving boundaries are often a source of conflict, and this is to be expected, especially in parent-child relationships, but poor communication doesn't have to be the norm.

A short cooking therapy session with "Adjustment Avocado Toast" could help either party to identify underlying feelings and express them thoughtfully. When you reinvent the way you share your concerns or even mandates in a way that someone can hear, everyone wins.

Ingredients

2 slices thin bread
1 very ripe avocado

2 slices tomato
Salt and pepper

Session Instructions

1. Think about any communication you've been having lately that feels thin, like your slices of bread. Notice the crust, too, which will represent the encircling of firmly held beliefs, at this point not ready to change. It's not always easy to change our style of speaking to

others to get our points across. Like our styles, the slices of bread are formed but not likely to hold the weight of "new thoughts." They need a slight change. And that's why we're here, isn't it? For even a slight change.

2. Turn on the toaster and commit to the catalyst of change that heat provides. Add your two slices.

3. Meanwhile, rinse the avocado, but don't rinse and repeat; just rinse once and tell yourself it's done. Take a mindful and concrete moment to note that no one responds well to being told the same thing over and over again and in the same way.

4. Make a shallow, circular cut around the avocado. Do you know the expression *Words cut deeper than a knife*? Resolve to use fewer sharp words and a softer tone with others and to cut less deep.

5. Notice the difference between the hard outer rind and the cool, green softness inside. The outside is hard and bumpy and dark. The inside is light and malleable. This represents opening up to change and taking your old style of speaking to a softer, lighter, and less rigid state.

6. Notice the obvious pit. No doubt this is the pit in your stomach when your thoughts create a style of communicating that's ineffective or, even worse, causes you or someone else to become frustrated or angry. TAKE IT OUT! Yes, at the "core" of the avocado is the chance for you to change how you feel and act. Saying the same thing over and over in the same way and getting little or no results is "the pits."

7. Using an everyday spoon, scoop the soft avocado out of its shell and into a bowl. I use the term *everyday* purposely. This new way of thinking takes practice,

and you may need to try it every day. Now mash the pulp with a fork or the back of the spoon, bringing it to an even softer and now spreadable consistency. As you think about changing the texture, identify your own style as either guarded (still in the shell), closed off (pit not removed), or still a bit hard (premashed in the bowl). Try something new so that you and your speech or body language are more manageable and malleable (adjusted and softened as necessary.). Take a mindful moment to think about this, and ask yourself honestly which description fits right now.

8. When the toast is ready, remove it and place it on a plate. As you spread the soft avocado onto the two slices, think about two ways or two places or two relationships where you can change what you say and how you say it. This applies even to self-talk. Sometimes we all say "I can't," but we can change that to "In the past, I never used to . . ." Do you see the difference? Slight changes in how we speak open up conversations and make challenges easier to contemplate.

9. Place a slice of tomato on each slice of toast. If you don't care for tomato, just look at the slices and remember the metaphor that tomatoes don't look done. The gelatinous insides seem as if they have a long way to go before they're done, like they're still evolving, just like evolving communication techniques.

10. Sprinkle salt and pepper to taste, and as you do so, imagine new and different sentences or styles of communicating. Practice out loud if possible both now and later. When you take a bite out of your "Adjustment Avocado Toast," imagine how satisfying it will be to be

heard and the possibilities that may ensue. Remember, when you speak differently, people respond differently; it's that simple.

TO GO

In this lesson, you've:

- Started out with a "thin" grasp on how to add new communication skills and adjust your way of speaking to others or to yourself.
- Heated things up for change and taken notice so that you're able to hold new ideas on your plate.
- Examined your current ways and whether or not they're working and given real effort and thought to a new or changing way of speaking, acting, or being.
- Thought about actual ways to be heard more clearly and not continually employ entrenched methods.
- Spread some different ideas so that now you can actually test them out. It's likely that changing some of your ways will have others surprised and listening in a way they previously haven't.

EASY RIDER: Cod With a Side of Clarity

When you're working through important issues, it's imperative to focus on being as clear as possible. For example, children need to learn their parents' nonnegotiable and firm tone. A boss will respond best if you calmly outline and highlight your contributions. And when your neighbor's pit bull keeps escaping from their yard, a conciliatory tone has a better chance of achieving your goals than threats to call the sheriff. When you're being unheard, a new way of communicating may be needed. Toward that end, I've created "Cod With a Side of Clarity."

Ingredients

½ pound cod (or other thin whitefish such as sole or tilapia)

1 tomato, chopped and seeded

1 cup leeks, white and green parts, chopped

½ cup yellow or orange bell pepper, chopped

2 tablespoons minced garlic

½ cup Italian breadcrumbs

½ cup plain baked potato chips

½ cup Parmesan cheese, grated

3 tablespoons butter, melted

Session Instructions

1. Lightly spray a sheet pan or cookie pan with nonstick spray. This is our first metaphor for thinking about communication patterns that have stuck with us for too long but we'd do well to have slide away. Take a minute and imagine one scenario where the way you communicated did not help you get you what you wanted.

2. Rinse the fish and think about washing away old styles that don't work. Remember the metaphor for rinse-and-repeat? We are definitely breaking that pattern by rinsing off old styles. Lay the fish aside on a cutting board, not yet on the pan.

3. Chopping vegetables can bring purpose and order. Chances are that when we speak "off the cuff" or speak from "reaction," our thoughts and words can tumble out in all sorts of shapes. Chopping uniformly has the

opposite effect. It's orderly and measured. Use this task to remind you to respond intentionally. A measured cadence will always have more impact than an emotional rant.

4. As you seed the tomatoes, think of planting new ways to address goals that have eluded you, and perhaps even imagine a new way of posturing a request or an idea. Take a mindful moment to also really think about a way you've communicated with yourself that might be ineffective, such as *It's too hard* or *I'm not up to the task*. Comedian George Carlin joked that tomatoes don't look like they're done yet because they look as if they're still in the "larvae" stage (Carlin & Urbisci, 1996). Embrace and believe in your own ability to evolve.

5. Chop the leeks and notice that they are a "sweet onion." Leeks sweeten as they cook. You may have something slightly unpleasant that can also result in a sweet end. Aren't leeks a little bit like life, then? We are always managing the sharp moments but hopefully also counting the sweet ones. This reminds us to be balanced and, in terms of communication, sends the message that we can address tough subjects in a way that's not heard only negatively.

6. I love the yellow pepper here, mostly for color, as a reminder that changing the way you communicate doesn't mean you have to be bland. You're allowed to be emphatic, even colorful, and to use your own style, as long as it's getting you the results you want. When it comes to self-talk, I encourage you to be colorful and strong. "I'm capable!" "I can do it!" "I'll succeed!"

7. Add the minced garlic and think about a way to "not mince words" but still use the lessons from all three

vegetables. As you combine everything, think about trying out new styles of communicating but still getting your point across. Perhaps you'll smile as you speak. Maybe you'll add some sweetness to your tone. Perhaps your words will be more measured. Just try on a new method in private till it feels like a fit. Think about a new suit. At first it might feel different from anything you've ever worn, but the important thing is that it fits and you feel comfortable wearing it.

8. Layer the vegetables onto the sheet pan in a shape that will accommodate the piece or pieces of fish. The vegetables make a base. How perfect is this? You've created a base for a new behavior and shaped your thoughts in a way that can be heard by others. Take a moment to appreciate the work you've done and can do going forward.

9. Combine the crumbs, chips, and cheese. Right now, you can think of these as old ways of communicating, styles that were formerly just loose bits and pieces with no real thought or purpose or craft, just hard chips and crumbs. They weren't bound together with thoughtful intent. We've been changing that.

10. Melt the butter in a microwave-safe dish and once again think about softening or melting any harsh style that causes others to "turn off." As you add the melted butter (softened style) to the hard crumbs, see how it starts to bring it all together and make a firmer paste. This is what happens when you melt old ways and firm up a new combination of skills.

11. Top the fish with the now-firm crumb mixture and think about topping off what we've discussed in this

session. Think about cementing or sealing in a new way of shaping your thoughts in the future. Although the recipe is "Cod With a Side of Clarity," the clarity is both the side and the main course.

12. Pop the fish into the oven and bake for approximately twenty minutes. You want to see the top browned; the "change in color" mirrors the changes you've made in thought and the actual changes you're going to try going forward. When you cut into the fish, you'll be able to actually see all of the steps in this session come together in one bite. That's a great morsel of clarity about what you say and how you say it, to yourself and others.

TO GO

Here are some reminders for you as you consider your experience from this session:

1. Remember to "unstick" old, unproductive ways and reorder styles that aren't working for you. Break the pattern of rinse-and-repeat.
2. Sweeten any harshness and find a way to "not mince words" but still get your point across.
3. Shape and use new methods as a base going forward, and continue to melt or soften any hard parts in how you speak to yourself or others.
4. Seal in and top off these new ways going forward.

Revisit this session to remind yourself whenever you need "a side of clarity."

SCENIC DRIVE: Think Twice Baked Potatoes

Let's talk a bit about technology and what can happen when we send texts that don't convey our true emotions. I know one mother-in-law who misstepped when her future daughter-in-law told her the name of her new niece. *Morgan Fisher* she texted. The mother-in-law texted back, jokingly, or so she thought, *Wow! A law firm!* Perhaps not the best response, but if it had been in person, her daughter-in-law would have also seen her smile and affect and heard the immediate phrase that followed, which was *So excited for them.*

This example doesn't even begin to address all that can go wrong with mistakenly sent texts or unseen texts, which can literally ruin relationships. We won't address "best texting" here but rather just offer a cautionary tale about what you do or don't put in writing.

A friend of mine, Dante, who had been a successful salesman for a medical device company, received an email that his company had been sold. Within a week, he was contacted, again by email, by the new director of his division, who was located in another state. The email seemed cold and unwelcoming and detailed new quotas that Dante felt were concerning. He shared with me that he didn't agree with the boss's business practices or the company's new mandates. For six months, Dante kept his feelings to himself, afraid for his job if he protested but concerned about the fallout for people he would never know. He considered being a whistleblower but wasn't sure his concerns were significant enough and "knew" that would be the end of his career because, as he said, who would ever hire him? His manager consistently led with threats such as "I want you to be afraid. My job is on the line, and that means yours is too." Over time, Dante ended up on Xanax and with a tremor he claimed was new. Both his manager's communication style and his internal communication were playing out as toxic. I knew we'd be unable to change his manager's way of communicating, but I thought Dante could change his self-talk and one of the ways to address it would be this cooking therapy session below.

If you're dealing with a tough situation where you're receiving toxic communication or even if you might just be making yourself toxic with negative self-talk, this session is for you. I named this recipe "Think Twice Baked Potatoes," because you'll have several moments to think twice about how you feel and/or act.

Ingredients

1 Idaho or russet potato
1 teaspoon olive oil
½ cup chicken stock
1 teaspoon butter

1 tablespoon grated Parmesan cheese
½ teaspoon paprika

Session Instructions

1. Preheat the oven to 450 degrees. Think about whether you are already at high heat in terms of feeling angry or frustrated so that you don't need to heat up anymore. There will be an opportunity to lower that heat, but first you need to acknowledge whether you're there.

2. Wash the potato and think about clearing your head. You've got a lot that you've held on to and taken in, but as you clear the dirt off the potato, this is a mindful

first step to begin clearing out what's been "dumped" on you.

3. Now take a fork and prick the potato two or three times so you can let the steam out while it bakes. Take a deep, cleansing breath and visualize letting some of the steam go. If you don't let negative feelings out properly, they are likely to come out in all the wrong ways. If the potato bursts instead of cooking evenly, you will be left with a huge mess. The same is true for keeping too much inside yourself. Eventually it can come out in ways that can create a potentially irreparable mess!

4. Take the teaspoon of oil in your hands and rub it all over the potato. Let's think about softening the outer layer of the potato and the inner layer of you. Everyone makes better decisions when they've had a chance to soften. This step does double duty, however, because when the potato is done, it will have a thicker skin, and that's also what you need when you're on the receiving end of toxic communication.

5. Place the potato on a rack in the oven and set a timer for forty-five minutes. While you wait, I want to tell you "the jack story." A man gets a flat tire on a rural highway. He calls for a tow truck. While he waits, he begins to think about how much the mechanic is going to charge him to tow him or to change the tire, and he begins to get agitated. He knows that the mechanic has him in a vulnerable spot and will overcharge him. He gets more worked up thinking about it. He tells himself that the mechanic will probably charge him for the tow, the change, and also the tire. He is getting really angry. *Then*, he thinks to himself, *that crooked mechanic is going to charge me for gas, and probably even to use the jack!* He gets so worked up that by the

time the mechanic arrives, he runs out of his car and goes right up to him and yells, "No way I'm going to pay you for the jack!"

Do you see what can happen when we catastrophize? In "the jack story," we never even get to meet the mechanic, who may not be a bad guy or overcharge at all. The only things we can deal with and process are actual facts and then our emotions toward them.

6. Remove the potato from the oven and notice how the skin is now hard and a bit crackly. Visualize that as the bad communication that's been coming at you but also as your thicker skin to handle it. Despite the hard shell, when you squeeze gently, there will be some give, letting you know that the potato is fully cooked. This is exactly how you will begin to feel now if you let the hard shell go; you'll have some flexibility in thought and words, and you'll have some "give" in your responses and be able to pause before you react. Let the potato pause too. Let it cool for a few minutes as you compel yourself to have the ability do the same. "Let cool" is a wonderful metaphor that you can always use and take with you.

7. Once the potato is cool enough to handle, use a sharp knife to slice it in half.

Can you think about that two ways? First, let's slice some perspective into what's going on. You can't change what others do, but you certainly can choose to filter what you take in so it isn't black mold, just annoying dust. This is a true "think twice" moment. Second, with two halves, there's an opportunity to imagine one half as negativity and the other as sunshine.

8. Scoop the negative half into a bowl. Get it all out and leave only the skin as a shell. Now scoop the positive

side into the bowl and think about it covering and dissolving the negative. Truly imagine the positive dissolving the negative and internalize that image. Now add the softened butter and chicken stock to the bowl and mix. Continue to think about all negative feelings being overpowered by other inner ingredients.

9. Once mixed, return the potato mixture to the skins. This is an important tangible step for returning positive feelings to your own skin.

10. Top the potato halves with Parmesan cheese and paprika. Now that you've been able to breathe through the hurt feelings and are thoughtful about how you choose to feel and/or respond, think of the cheese and paprika as the external steps you'd like to take. Maybe you will speak your mind, send an email or text, or simply plan.

11. Return the potatoes to the oven for ten more minutes to warm. During this time you can warm up to your new ideas. Then put the potatoes under the broiler for one to two minutes to sear—and of course sear in your new feelings—but watch them carefully so the cheese doesn't burn. Now you will have two halves with positive feelings going forward but also a hard crust to withstand cruelty and a hard top so that the cruelty doesn't seep in.

TO GO

Here are some reminders for you as you process this session:

- Remember to soften your instinct for reacting instead of responding and let the steam out before you do.

- Slice options into your plan when negative communications occur, and scoop positive thoughts onto the negative ones.
- Melt and dilute the urge to internalize negative self-talk or others' toxic messages.
- Warm up to the image of having a skin thick enough to withstand destructive communications and thoughtfully plan your next moves, both internal and external.
- As always, you can't control others, but you can decide how you choose to feel and react.

After-Dinner Mint

Remember, most traditional therapy sessions do not create breakthroughs in one session but rather after rapport has been established, comfort has been reached, and some of the thoughts and questions have had time to "marinate." This can happen days, weeks, and months later.

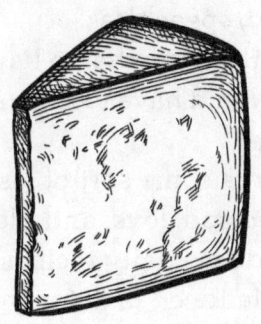

Chapter Twelve

Cooking Therapy for Couples, Families, and Groups

Several years ago, even before I was a clinician and the Sous Therapist™, I was at a playdate for my son. We were preparing lunch for the kids, and one of the four-year-olds turned to his mom and asked, "You always loved me, right, Mommy?"

"Yes, of course, sweetie."

"You loved me even before I was born?"

We all chuckled as she answered, "Yep, even before you were born."

"Even when I was in your tummy?"

"Yes, yes, even when you were in my tummy."

"And you loved me before that, when I was still food?"

Wait, what?

We all just stared, speechless.

Imagine a child thinking that to have gotten into his mom's tummy, she would have to have *eaten* him! Now that was amusing.

And yet, isn't there some sort of lesson here about the connection between food, love, and life? These days my Instagram feed sends me daily recipes for "Marry Me Chicken," "Marry Me Rice," or "Marry Me Veal Milanese." The food/love/cooking connection is no coincidence. It was only a matter of time before the process of cooking became a tool in the journey to mental health.

When it comes to food, everyone has a memory of a perfect meal that somehow has never been duplicated, even with the same ingredients or a visit to the same restaurant. Upon further exploration, you often learn that while it may have been delicious chicken scarpariello or key lime pie, more than likely the company was special and the emotions, anything from camaraderie to peace to lust, contributed to the perfectly cooked pasta or "best bite ever."

In fact, I know one couple who reminisce about a "late-night snack," as they describe the date where they knew their relationship was getting serious. Jillian, a thirty-six-year-old woman who was undergoing fertility treatments, was referred to me at the women's wellness center where I worked. She was becoming increasingly anxious and depressed from the multiple injections, egg retrievals, and evaluations of egg viability as well as three failed implantations. She was working full-time and was physically and emotionally exhausted as well as experiencing mood swings, likely from the hormones as well as the stress and schedule. Fortunately, her husband was supportive and accompanied her to therapy whenever she asked. They were the epitome of a loving young couple. I remember a session where they both told the same story about when they were dating.

"The eggs at that diner were better than any we'd ever had. We both wondered if they might be raising chickens in the yard!"

In downtown Passaic, New Jersey? Not likely. But the feeling of the moment made the meal special. And the couple moved in together just a month after that meal! Our connection to the thing that nurtures us, nourishes us, and keeps us alive is indelible.

And it's not just taste. Even the smell of food brings back memories of love. For me, fried onions announce that my grandmother must be in the kitchen, even though she's been gone for forty years, and tarragon will always remind me of a time in my life when I felt challenged, loved, and ultimately supported. It was a tarragon chicken salad kind of summer.

A cooking therapy session can help you explore any and all relationships in your life. Sometimes we know exactly why we're at odds with the people in our lives, but at other times we need a little excavating.

Parents of young children can begin to acclimate their kids to expressing emotions by having them join in a cooking therapy session for just a few moments, or as long as they'd like. Families with older kids may know that the hormonal fallout and varying emotional extremes of that life stage are developmentally appropriate but still incredibly confusing and often all-consuming to navigate. This is a perfect time to create a family cooking session that is nonconfrontational and lighthearted in tone. Not only will it be illuminating for all, but it will reap rewards in terms of mutual understanding and family time.

In addition to improving relationships with core family members, cooking therapy can help with relational issues involving partners, siblings, parents, or even coworkers.

Cooking Therapy for Couples, Groups, and Families

The bulk of my clinical experience has been with individuals. That said, when I was a school social worker, I created many small groups for youngsters from ages ten to seventeen, depending on the school where I was based. I was a member of the child study teams at three elementary schools and two high schools over the course of my school social work career. During that time, I participated in many individual education plan (IEP) meetings, family meetings, and annual reviews. In these meetings it was determined whether a child qualified for special education and, if so, what kind. At the time, possible classifications centered primarily on intellectual disability, speech impairment, or emotional disturbance. A child that met the qualifications for any classification would often receive educational support in the form of extra tutoring, other resources or therapy, and, at times, small-group instruction in a separate classroom.

Later in my private practice and in my work with substance abuse and psychiatric treatment facilities as well as for the state of New Jersey, I had the privilege of meeting with parents, siblings, teens, therapists, and psychiatrists and learned much more about family and couple relationships. I am not an expert in these areas, as they require additional education and a certification called licensed marriage and family therapist (LMFT). However, I do know that cooking therapy can address so many of the familial and relational issues that occur.

Finally, just before COVID, I began to receive requests to provide cooking therapy to many groups and organizations from wildly varying places, like Bloomingdale's and the IBD (Irritable Bowel Department) of Mount Sinai Hospital in New York City as well as religious organizations and book clubs.

Through my work with so many different populations, I became experienced at implementing cooking therapy with couples, groups, and families. In this chapter I will impart a "taste" of some of the sample sessions appropriate for each of these groups.

Families

Research proves that community is an essential component of longevity and happiness. What does that mean for today's families? Many of our workdays are longer in terms of online connectivity, even though some of us are working remotely or in hybrid models. As we and our children get more connected to tech and less to family and community, isolation is abundant.

When I was working in the substance abuse and co-occurring disorders field, I had the opportunity to visit a renowned treatment center in Connecticut and participate in an activity in their family program called the balloon game. Several of us stood in a circle, and we each had a balloon, but only one person had a green balloon. We were instructed to play the balloon game by keeping all the balloons from falling on the floor but were told that no matter what, we could not let the green balloon drop. As you can imagine, craziness ensued, trying to keep all the balloons in the air but especially the green one. Adults were lurching and lunging and generally falling all over the place. All the colored balloons eventually fell to the floor as we managed to keep the green one in the air till the whistle blew. Here was the major, tangible, and concrete message: Ask yourself what has fallen to the floor when one person or activity is so much more important than anything else and takes up more of your time? What is getting lost in terms of family time or connection? Where are all the other balloons?

Additionally, bringing a family into balance is a complicated task. A longtime model used in family therapy is systems theory developed by Ludwig von Bertalanffy. In its simplest terms, systems theory states that when one piece in a system changes, all the others must change to accommodate the shift. A family is a system. A shift in the system requires all to shift. This refers not only to the one family member who may be "taking more of their share" but to the vested interest all the family members have in keeping things the same, even if the system is suffering. Change is hard. In cooking therapy, we can tease out many of the pieces and players in the family system in a fun, enjoyable, connected, and enlightening way. Parents and teens will learn about themselves while also partaking in "community."

Let's give it a try with one recipe. I've named it "Tune In and Talk to Me Tacos." Using this recipe in a family session allows for all participants to make choices, own them without judgment, and move out of their comfort zone by trying new things. Families may learn things about each other's likes and dislikes, regrets, and aspirations and gain information that they previously didn't know. Knowledge and expression, which are two of the features of "Tune In and Talk to Me Tacos," are the result in this recipe and, because it's done through the medium of food choice, may create the beginning of change in the system in a way that can be less jarring and more tolerated.

Tune In and Talk to Me Tacos

With families so scheduled and moving in so many different directions, it's a challenge to entice everyone to the table, but tacos seem to do the trick: easy, cost-effective, and fun! I say *olé*! This recipe and activity works for all ages, including young children. For this session it's essential that all tech, including parents' cell phones, is turned off and put away, optimally in another room. Remember to have everyone participate in the cooking therapy rules:

- Respect the space
- Name the recipe (I've done it here for you)
- Take stock of what you've brought to the table
- Be present
- Wash your hands before you begin

Children and teens may have trouble "tuning in" to what they've brought to the table. As a substitute, ask each family member to name one thing that brings them joy. This will set the tone for participation and self-reflection. Parents should model tuning in by naming their own version of taking stock or being present.

Ingredients

1 prepackaged taco box that offers both hard and soft taco shells

1 pound each of two ground meats (or veggie sub), such as beef, chicken, or turkey

2 packages (8 ounces) grated cheese of your choice

10 toppings of your choice (e.g., tomatoes, lettuce, onions, green or black olives, salsa, sour cream, scallions, guacamole, chocolate!)

Session Instructions

1. Ask everyone to choose either a hard or soft taco. Highlight the fact that everyone is different and that's okay. Ask each person to name one thing about them that is different from other family members. It may be that one is an early bird and another a night owl. Someone likes

sports and another likes art. For young children, it may be chocolate versus vanilla. The important thing is for everyone to go around and say something they like and for each person to be supported. Parents can guide the topics.

2. Now have everyone choose whether they want chicken or beef (or one of the two choices you've provided.). You may already know the answer, but this is a tangible therapy that cements connection. Having everyone say their choice just affirms that all choices are acceptable and welcome. Some discussion and banter may occur. Parents should direct it to be positive and affirming. Now go around and have each family member say something positive about themselves, such as "I'm a good friend," "I'm smart," "I'm kind," or "I'm creative."

3. Parents, place the meats in two separate pans and simmer. Ask each family member to notice how the "raw" meat sizzles and smells good as it turns from one substance that is unhealthy to eat into another that is delicious. Older children can have a turn stirring the pan. Discuss "stirring in change" and evolving. Go around the room and ask each member to name a way they've evolved. This is a difficult task for some. Keep this activity fun and supportive by saying, "That's okay." Parents should model this by highlighting a change they've made but don't pressure children or teens if they're stuck. Believe it or not, they will think about this later and it will have a benefit.

4. Parents, once the meat is cooked, drain the fat from the meats and highlight draining something from themselves or the family that doesn't benefit the "dish." Stay positive. Parents may say "I wish I could be home more" or "I'd like to spend more time together" or "I wish we

weren't all in so much of a hurry" or "I hate that I snap sometimes." It's up to you how disclosing you'd like to be. Kids may say different or unexpected things. They may say nothing. Be supportive. Once again, family sessions do not always seem powerful in the moment but reap rewards later.

5. Add the seasoning. In this session, seasoning will be a metaphor for aspiring. Have each family member cite a challenge or desire. Parents may say, "I'd like to make more time for a hobby." Kids may say, "I want to take tennis lessons." If anyone is feeling insightful, they may state, "I'd like to work on being more patient." Parents can model healthy aspiring, but remember to keep the activity fun. Sometimes a child or teen may be especially expressive. Make sure to listen, respond, and validate any thoughts and keep other family members from devaluing this child through habit (remember systems theory?) or discomfort. Support that child and move on. Dynamics between siblings can be difficult to manage if one is continually surly. Remember this may be a pattern or defense mechanism and try hard not to react.

6. Have everyone take their taco and fill it. Filling is a great metaphor. Once again, name one or two things that "fill you up." Help younger children talk about enjoying school or a subject or a friend. Encourage teens to dig a little deeper than just topical items like "I like music" by modeling. Parents might say, "I feel good about myself when I finish a project or a colleague compliments me." Or say, "When I hear a certain song, I feel inspired." A good discovery prompt is the question *What about it?* So if your child says, "I like basketball," follow with "What about it?" Even if

they don't answer, this response models thinking and reflecting.

7. Sprinkling cheese is the perfect metaphor for sprinkling compliments. If a family member doesn't want cheese, they can still participate in this step. Go around the room and have each person give a compliment to every family member. Sometimes you will have a child or teen with a case of the *I don't know*s. That's okay. Simply say, "We'll come back to you, and if you think of one later, let us know." You'll be surprised, because they often do.

8. Toppings are going to model not only supporting differences but also stepping out of your comfort zone. Ask each family member to make their perfect taco with all of the toppings they like. This is a good time to reflect on how differences don't have to be distancing but instead can be connecting as you all enjoy a meal together. If possible, for a second taco, ask each member—including young children—to try one topping they haven't tried before (or even switch from their chosen shell). Parents should model this, even if it's done with playful grimaces or funny protests. This is an opportunity to model trying new things and growth and can also be extremely fun if everyone does it. Even if some members won't finish the taco or they pull the new pieces out, the message of expanding horizons sticks.

9. Everyone should participate in the cleanup. Use this time to talk about the session and what worked or didn't, or simply enjoy being a family who shared a meal that wasn't hurried or interrupted and explored some feelings and emotions. Family cooking therapy is especially exponential, meaning it can reap rewards in other areas.

Not only will everyone think about the session itself, but the process of self-exploration has been initiated and developed. This session will have "legs," and both children and teens will often ask for a repeat.

TO GO

Here are some pieces of advice to remember about this session, or any other cooking therapy family sessions you'd like to try:

- Keep remarks about the session low-key and casual. Statements such as "That was fun" or "Loved that" are great. Although I sometimes like to leave worksheets with clients, I do not suggest a worksheet for family sessions, as most kids have enough of those at school.
- If you have that very insightful teen who wants to discuss family issues more deeply, be available and receptive. This does not have to involve everyone once the session is done. Remember that even those teens who professed to get nothing out of the experience will absorb the message that "tuning in" and connecting is a family value.

Groups

Another therapist utilizing cooking therapy is Julie Ohana from Michigan. Recently, she was quoted in CNN talking about using cooking therapy in groups. Julie says, "Culinary arts therapy can also make the most out of group sessions. If you're with the group, part of the magic that I like to think happens is in the interaction with the people that you're with. You're really learning to communicate and problem-solve with others in a way that you don't really find in other situations" (Lee, 2019). I couldn't agree more! Whenever I'm asked to do a presentation or demonstration with a group, the feedback is amazing. It's no wonder that so many treatment centers and programs are beginning to catch on. We'll talk more about cooking therapy with groups in another chapter.

Every single time I've presented and guided a group of people through a cooking therapy session, someone has had an epiphany, that *aha* moment, and while many are positive, some are not, just as with Nora from the Introduction, who realized her marriage was beyond repair. I've had participants become upset, cry, or become angry as a way to combat the feeling of vulnerability that may occur.

It's important to be aware of this and discuss it with the participants in advance. Everyone needs to know and feel that whatever feelings come up, there is support and they are in a safe place. I suggest you become comfortable and skilled by tackling most or all of the sessions in this book, and then you can give it a try with "Don't Be Chicken Chicken." This is a quick and easy recipe for evaluating where you are and/or where you'd like to be that lends itself to a lunch or dinner and shouldn't ruffle too many chicken feathers. I've used this recipe with book clubs and always get positive feedback. Remember to remove technology from the room and that my universal cooking therapy rules apply.

- Respect the space
- Name the recipe (I've done it here for you)

- Take stock of what you've brought to the table
- Be present
- Wash your hands before you begin

Don't Be Chicken Chicken

A common thread in many groups I've presented to is the struggle to know what to do "next." By this I mean instances where the kids are more independent, or the company had layoffs, or "I've always wanted to _____ (fill in the blanks), but I don't know where or how to start." For that reason, I created "Don't Be Chicken Chicken." The name is meant to "prompt" you up, because I've been there and countless of clients have been there, and I know that every new move starts with a little step or push and so I hope this cooking therapy session gives that to you. My rules of group therapy still apply: Confidentiality and kindness live here. What's said in the room stays in the room. You're more than welcome to switch out chicken with eggs, in which case you can call the recipe "Which Came First?"

Ingredients

1 package romaine or Bibb lettuce, prewashed

1–2 rotisserie chickens, depending on size of group (or 6–8 hard-boiled eggs)

1 package celery, organic if possible

½ cup mayonnaise per person, any kind

Session Instructions

1. Remove the lettuce from the package and place one or two leaves on your plate. This is the first layer of a new

mindset or move. It's where you've been or possibly a metaphor for a new layer of you. The lettuce is bright green and fresh and crisp, just like a new idea.

2. Each person should take a wing or leg of the chicken, like you're flying or walking off into a new adventure. State your desire or wish either out loud or to yourself, whichever feels more comfortable. Take a moment to solidify it.
   If using hard-boiled eggs, each person should hold the egg up (like Mustafa in *The Lion King*) and do the same.

3. Peel the skin off the leg or wing or the shell off the hard-boiled egg. It's not that easy, and of course peeling back what may be holding you back is not easy either. Do your best, and it's okay if a little skin remains. That's kind of like life, right? We move forward, but a little fear and doubt remain. Totally normal. However, if using eggs, simply recognize that this happens, but do remove all of the shell.

4. Remove meat from the wings and legs, adding peeled meet from the breasts or thighs. Whether using chicken or eggs, place them on a cutting board and chop. As you do, think of chopping old doubts and fears away. Anything holding you back. Name them out loud or to yourself—for example, logistics, finances, fear of failure, other people's stifling words, your own negative self-talk, even past failures. Chop that all away. Then place the "pure" chicken or egg, with any hard parts removed, in a bowl.

5. Each person washes one celery stalk purposefully. Think about the ambition you stated out loud or to yourself and wash away even more self-doubt.

6. Now chop the celery into bite-size pieces and commit to "chopping in" confidence, faith, and conviction that you

are worthy and capable. The bite-size pieces represent making moves that are small at first and manageable. Place the chopped celery in the bowl.

7. What will keep all this conviction together? You've taken a nagging feeling and peeled away negative self-talk to reveal an actual desire. You've chopped away self-doubt and chopped in conviction and maybe even a plan. Now let's seal it together. Add the mayonnaise to the bowl and mix together everything you've done today.

8. Place the chicken salad or egg salad on your lettuce layer, and sprinkle salt and pepper to taste to symbolize sprinkling in a new view or resolve. Say, "Lettuce" (let us) remember, 'Don't Be Chicken Chicken.'" You're allowed to smile!

> *Note:* Another way I've run groups is by pairing up individuals and having them go through the steps but share their feelings about each step semi-privately with a partner. Again, this requires a trained therapist, and the rules of group therapy apply.

Couples

A cooking therapy session with a couple is almost always diagnostic, as you learn a lot about couples by how they interact when preparing a dish together.

One partner chops vegetables in perfect slices while the other simply chops in a random way with slices of different sizes. How they react to each other over even this small task is illuminating and can be reflected back by the therapist so that the couple can generalize it to their relationship.

One professes to be totally uncomfortable in the kitchen while the other smiles with confidence. Will the "uncomfortable" partner let the other do all the work? How does the "working" partner feel and act about doing so? Again, the opportunities for discussion of patterns and habits and feelings are abundant.

There may be a scenario where one partner looks expectant while the other checks their watch, isn't paying attention, or makes silly or irrelevant jokes. When this happens, the focused partner can feel frustrated or devalued while the distracted, joking partner may feel either that there's no problem or that, if there is, it belongs to the other person. I've seen it all.

There are so many things you can notice while doing couples cooking therapy, but it's important to have a productive session and not one that's damaging. For instance, if one partner is more kitchen savvy, there may be an imbalance of power, perceived or real. These are a few of the minefields you may encounter in a couples cooking therapy session. If a session becomes heated (between you two, not the food), pause and reflect and try to inject some fun into the activity. Let go of the clinical part and just cook together. If you're in traditional therapy, then bring the subject up at your next meeting.

The optimal way for a couples cooking therapy session to work would be if both of you have read most or all of this book and joyfully want to try a recipe as equal members of a team in pursuit of relationship revelations. To that end, I've provided you with "Couples Contemplations Crunch." This recipe is not for you to fix anything but rather to help you explore and share your feelings. Remember to remove technology from the room and that my universal cooking therapy rules apply.

- Respect the space
- Name the recipe (I've done it here for you)
- Take stock of what you've brought to the table
- Be present
- Wash your hands before you begin

Couples Contemplations Crunch

This recipe was originally passed on to me by my cousin Dena, but I've come to learn that most people are familiar with it despite not knowing the origin. A version made for the Jewish holiday of Passover uses matzo and is credited to Marcy Goldman.

Ingredients

Escort (or similar) crackers, enough to cover the bottom of an approximately 10 × 15 cookie sheet

1 cup (2 sticks) unsalted butter
1 cup firmly packed brown sugar
¾ cup semisweet, milk, or white chocolate chips

Session Instructions

1. Preheat the oven to 375 degrees. Take a mindful moment and together discuss how heat is a catalyst for change and how, while the heat will change the consistency of this dish, it can also change your relationship if you wish. If there are changes either of you would like to see, now is a time to mention them.
2. Line the baking sheet with parchment paper. This "crunch" is going to get sticky. We want the lessons to stick, the sharing to stick, but not so much that you can't discuss or modify it.

3. Starting at different ends, each of you may take the crackers and line the sheet with them. As you go, take turns mentioning three things you like or love about your partner. You need not state a feeling for every cracker, just as you go.

4. Continue to layer, and then each of you may state one thing, but only one, that feels missing or that you may be wanting in order for the relationship to "come together" more. Take a mindful moment to really listen. If you're not sure you understand, ask for further clarification. This is not a put-down or *you* statement, as in "You need to like sports." It's an *I* statement, such as "I wish we'd both take more walks together" or "I wish we'd be on our phones less."

5. Meet in the middle with your crackers, making sure the sheet pan is covered and making sure you understand each other's statements. Each of you may now place one final cracker and state how you might be able to meet the other's needs, based on their statement. Do not argue! Problem-solve or commit to giving the other's needs some attention.

6. In a heavy saucepan, combine the butter and brown sugar over medium heat until the mixture comes to a boil, stirring constantly. Talk about any issues that have been "boiling" but can be better served if stirred over a lower flame. This will take two to four minutes, just enough time to discuss but not to "overstir." Boil for three more minutes, stirring, and notice how the bubbles make it impossible to see the mixture clearly. Let that metaphor sit with you. When things are bubbling hot, they are unclear.

7. Take note that you are bringing the mixture almost to the hard-crack stage. It's worth exploring what issues

are so hot that the temperature rises to a point where nothing is malleable and each of you feels like you might just break. If these exist, put them out into the atmosphere so they can lose their inner seal and energy.

8. When ready, carefully pour the hot mixture over the crackers without upsetting them. Going forward, will you be able to do the same with issues concerning your relationship? In other words, can you still "pour your heart out" but in a way that doesn't have your partner going to pieces?

9. Place the sheet in the oven and immediately lower the temperature to 350 degrees. Wow, what a great visual for a discussion that may get too hot! If this happens to you, remember turning down the oven's temperature and turn down your own.

10. Bake for fifteen minutes, checking to see if the crunch is getting too brown or burnt. Check in with each other: How are you each doing and feeling? If you're too hot, lower the oven and yourselves to 325 degrees.

11. Remove the pan from the oven and immediately sprinkle chocolate chips over the crunch. This is a chance to sprinkle kind words over each other and to end the session on a positive note. Compliments, thanks, wonderful memories, and laughter can all be sprinkled onto the crunch at this time.

12. After five minutes, each of you may spread the chocolate out with a spatula and spread in all of the positive words you shared.

13. While still warm from the good feelings, break the crackers up into different sizes. The snap of the crunch could simulate hardness being snapped away or even signify that working on communication and sharing "is

a snap" in a cooking therapy session! Perhaps you might even "crack up" when you reminisce about the metaphors in this recipe.

14. Finally, place the crunch in the refrigerator and let it chill until set. Do the same with all the things you discussed. Let them chill for now, and now that they have that space, they are more likely to set. Then enjoy your "Couples Contemplations Crunch" together.

As you can see, cooking therapy has multiple applications that can impact the many relationships in your life. Now that you've had the opportunity to try cooking therapy with families, couples, and groups, let's take a look at the expansive and convenient ways cooking therapy can be used with your preferred ingredients or those you already have at hand.

Chapter Thirteen

Create Your Own Cooking Therapy Session

In this section of *Cooking as Therapy*, you will have the opportunity to create your own cooking therapy sessions based on the ingredients you have at hand or choose. For instance, if you want to make your favorite banana bread that uses bananas, walnuts, sugar, and flour, you can simply find those ingredients in this section and the processes they represent, and you're on your way to becoming your own sous therapist™.

We'll start with some metaphors that work for some of the most common cooking actions. These metaphors can be applied to whatever you cook. Then I'll move on to the ingredient list, which includes more tailored cooking therapy tips for each food group and item.

There are at least five samples in each category. Many of the entries can double if you have a similar item. For example, I've included cantaloupes, but if you have a similar melon or fruit with a bumpy rind and seeds, the process may be the same. The same might occur with yogurt and milk. If you tease out the metaphors in one, you can likely do the same with the other.

So delve into the categories below. They are ready for you whenever you decide to explore, uncover, change, or reflect, for yourself or your family.

Common Cooking Processes

Stirring

Patience: Whenever I think it's appropriate to infuse a metaphor for patience into a session, stirring does the trick. Whether the instructions say "stir till thick," "stir constantly," or "stir till bubbles form," patience is required. If you're someone who is not used to waiting, I suggest trying a recipe with instructions to stir and then thinking about something else while you do. You can use the time to try to resolve an issue in your head, but even better would be to think of a happy memory and let that play mentally. Try to reassociate waiting with something pleasurable. You could even sing a song or write a poem in your head. Stirring can be very calming and pleasurable. This can be a tool that can generalize to other moments in your life where patience is required.

Chopping

If you're struggling with an overwhelming sense of discord or feeling that something is wrong (or everything is wrong), chopping can be used in combination with many ingredients to sort it all out. For the most part, chopping is methodical and orderly. In cooking, no matter what recipe you prepare, chopping vegetables to the same approximate size is recommended, so it's rather purposeful. Reducing unmanageable feelings into one or two that can be addressed is often the main goal of therapy.

A fun way to think about the act of chopping would be to take note of the food show *Chopped*. The name applies to a contestant being removed or "chopped out." Slowly and carefully "chopping out" is a goal for taking a large, engulfing problem or feeling and breaking it down into a "piece" or "pieces" you can name and address and remove.

Frying

I think frying is great for excavating intense emotions, and not just because it sounds like "crying" (well, at least to me). The actual act of frying involves heating up oil and transforming a substance from loose to hard or hard to soft. It's about the change and the sizzle and the heat and the sound and the chance to think about change. Change might mean something tangible or emotional. It might simply be a chance to change your mood.

If you're "deep frying," then by all means go deep. Frying often involves holding on to a pan and taking control. No matter what is being fried, there is usually a noticeable smell. If you are angry or upset, if you feel that something has to change, frying can mirror that and both release the intensity and firm up your resolve. You can also look at the food you're frying and see a change, so the metaphor is visual.

Also, being fried means being tired. So once again, if you need to affirm the feeling that you're tired of something and done with it, frying is for you.

Boiling

Like frying, boiling is one of those methods that can help you identify and excavate feelings of anger, frustration, and stress. Bringing items to a boil requires intense heat, and eventually you will see the evidence that something is boiling with bubbles, which is often kind of how you feel when negative feelings "bubble up." So it's actually a good representation for a mindful moment, acknowledging the level of intensity of those feelings. We never go past the boiling point in cooking, right? And that's a metaphor for learning there's a limit to your feelings and no need to go further or act in any way. Sitting with feelings is tough, but eventually you realize that until you turn down the heat, you can't see into the pot. The boiling water is not clear, right? It's filled with chaotic bubbles that occlude what's inside. That's kind of like you if you're boiling mad. But as soon as you take down the heat, the water becomes clearer, and there's your message: Calm leads to clarity; chaos leads to confusion.

Maybe your feelings built up a long time before you got to your boiling point. Perhaps next time when you have feelings that are snowballing, you can share or address them before they get that hot. We all can feel, even physically, when tension and frustration and anger are building up inside. Try breathing, taking a walk to clear your head, or simply walking away from an increasingly toxic situation before you get to the boiling point.

Coring and Seeding

Removing items that are buried or unseen, like cores, seeds, or pits, is a great opportunity to get to the heart of a problem and plan to name what's going on "inside." I suggest that you take a moment to pause, look at what's physically coming out, like an apple core, tomato core, avocado pit, or cucumber seeds, and question whether anything is going on that you'd like to change or address. Also, removing cores and seeds is a wonderful process for facing secrets. Think about what happens if you leave a core in your pie, or the stems of a strawberry in your parfait. Uneatable. Secrets can be toxic. I'm not saying confessions are always good, you'll have to evaluate, but if something is buried that you can't reveal, open up to someone safe.

However, not everything in coring or seeding is about problems. You have wonderful inner qualities and a core that's solid and strong; this is a good time to take a moment to recognize and enjoy it. No doubt you've worked hard to achieve a sense of sturdiness that sustains you. Use this process to affirm that you don't want to lose it and applaud yourself for even more than a minute!

Peeling

Peeling back, peeling away, peeling off. All of these expressions are about looking beneath the surface and discovering what's underneath, and that's exactly what peeling is for in cooking therapy. Many of us become comfortable going about our lives in the "skin we're in," even when we have nagging problems. It seems like a lot of work to look underneath. When we peel the skin off an apple or cucumber, what do we see? Softer, lighter, fresher food that is usually more malleable for the peeling. It's almost impossible to get real or express yourself when covered in a hard skin. Think about that the next time you peel. And if things are going well, enjoy thinking that there's no need to peel anything back, but always "keep your eyes peeled."

Sifting

Sifting provides a wonderful opportunity to obtain a perfect visual of any hard pieces that need to be taken out. What sort of hard pieces? Hard-and-fast rules or values that would benefit from examination, a hardened heart that has created discord in a relationship, a hard tone when you greet or interact with others at work or home.

Also, ask yourself to simply sift through your choices. Some have slid easily into place while others not so much.

Sifting through feelings is a wonderful tool to determine how you feel right now. Whether you make a pros-and-cons list or just commit to focusing, sifting should remind you that you deserve softness and not situations or people that give you "a hard time."

Heating

One of the mainstays of cooking therapy is "turning on the heat." We do this with our oven, our toaster, and our pots and pans, and always it is a metaphor for change. This change may not be monumental but simply a slight change in our readiness to entertain new thoughts and ideas and explore our self-talk, feelings, and behaviors. Heath is a catalyst for change; it will braise, boil, roast, fry, and crisp your food. Every time you turn on the heat, no matter the device, imagine integrating a readiness to see things in a new way.

Ingredient List

In the pages ahead you will find over one hundred common ingredients, broken down into eight familiar categories that you can incorporate into any cooking therapy session you choose.

Fruits

Cantaloupes/Melons

The whole fruit: Before you begin, hold the whole canta-loupe in your hands. Take a mindful moment and notice how it feels, bumpy and rather rough. Think about how it will feel to remove the rind and the toughness, smooth out some of the bumps, and get to the juiciness in life that should and can be yours.

    Seeds: When you cut the melon open and scoop out the seeds, ask yourself what you might be able to *remove* in your day-to-day routine that keeps you from scooping sweetness *into* your life. Also, look at all those seeds. Even if things are going well, they're a great symbol of how you can plant new ideas and behaviors to grow goodness at any time.

Berries (strawberries, blackberries, blueberries, raspberries, etc.)

The whole berry: I love when I'm making a pie, trifle, or smoothie that calls for multiple berries. Before I begin, I fill a glass bowl with blueberries, strawberries, blackber-ries, raspberries, and even kiwi and truly stop and stare for sixty seconds (it's not that easy to be so still, is it?) and breathe in the beauty. Even if you're just using one type of berry, try it. When you take a moment to enjoy the beauty of nature, the variety of colors and textures, you give yourself a gift. You can almost feel the calm starting from your forehead and melting down your body.

Appearance: Berries are almost always juicy, bursting with goodness, as you can intentionally try to be. They are basically round, which is a great prompt for not having rough edges, and usually brightly colored. How wonderfully aspirational to think of *colorful* as meaning having multiple interests and unique traits. Berries have small seeds, which is encouraging for little steps forward, and they do not have pits. Hooray! Pitless fruit is a great representation of having no "pits in your stomach," which means no secrets or unhelpful regrets.

Mangoes/Kiwis

Rind: I find mangoes hard to peel; how about you? And then it's a lot of work for a relatively small amount of fruit. But boy, if that fruit is ripe, how delicious, and you know instantly that it was worth the work. Some people are like that; you don't get to know them as easily at first, but they're worth it. This is a good time to ask yourself if you're surrounding yourself with people of quality, and not just "playful" friends and relatives who lack substance. When adding mango to a recipe, ask yourself if the people in your life are adding or subtracting to your mental health.

Bananas/Plantains

Peeling: I call bananas and plantains the honesty fruits. Don't lose the chance to do some major peeling back and looking inwardly at yourself. As you peel the fruit, think about how you show yourself to the world. It's a great time to ponder showing the world your real self, even with some bruises. I say way too often that I like my friends the way I like my bananas, with some bruises (flaws), because those totally unscathed yellow ones can be hard and hard to digest. Don't forget to show *yourself* yourself too. And love what's inside and underneath.

Create calm: If you cut up the peel and boil a banana or plantain in about two cups of water, it creates a calming drink called banana tea.

Apples/Pomegranates/Watermelons/Papayas

Seeds: I like apples for exploring those nagging little insecurities, worries, and doubts that we all have. Rather than one big pit, an apple has many small ones, as do the other fruits you can substitute here. You wouldn't eat those seeds, right? So why retain so many concerns and worries about things that you can't control or really don't matter? Scoop out those little seeds and think about letting go of all the little fears and troubles you can't change. Remember that often the only thing you can control about a situation is how you choose to feel or react.

Idioms: There are several idioms for apples. If you have a bad apple in your life, perhaps it's time to think about your relationships and how you like your friends or partners. Identify and think about how this person is affecting you and what you'd like to do about it. Also, what about being the "apple of your own eye"? That's right, another chance to love yourself. When it comes to a watermelon or papaya, in addition to scooping out little seeds or problems, think about how you might "take a slice out of life" in a new and positive way.

Tomatoes/Grapes

Appearance: Carlin's joke that tomatoes don't look like they're done yet because they look as if they're still in the "larvae" stage is one I use a lot during cooking therapy. I feel like I owe him a debt for those comments because they are almost too perfect as a metaphor for evolving! I feel the same way about grapes. The insides are gelatinous.

When you cook with tomatoes or slice grapes, notice how they seem to be still developing and remind yourself that evolving is key to growth. Also, remember that it's never too late to make a change or go for a goal.

Cooking: Next, it's true that tomatoes and grapes shrivel, especially when cooked at high heat. But we don't necessarily have to think of shriveling as the metaphor. We can look at shriveling and resolve not to! Ask yourself if there's an area in your life where you've "shrunk back" or been too timid or reticent. Have a mindful moment as you look at the shrunken fruits: delicious in the pan but not so much in life! Resolve to move forward just a bit, even gently, with confidence.

Vegetables

Cucumbers/Zucchini

These are one of the staples in my therapy pantry. They provide so many metaphors for a variety of self-evaluation.

Peeling: First, when you peel away the darkest part, it can represent uncovering newness in thought or change. The peel can represent the old skin you've been in, the one that just got comfy or familiar but wasn't empowering. Maybe you are not really who you are or want to be? As you get rid of it, do it purposefully. Throw it away with some vigor and ask, "What's left?" Not an empty space but a substantive and solid and cool fresh entity, aka you.

Slicing and chopping: Slice into the cucumber or zucchini and observe the green freshness and seeds. They represent hope and new thoughts or beginnings. Think about any fresh ideas or behaviors you'd like to plant in your life. When you chop these vegetables, whether into chunks or rounds, they can represent chances to look at parts of your life, like your career, family, or hobbies (chunks) or your personality traits (rounds). Whatever you choose, cucumbers have "lengthy" benefits.

Mushrooms

Chopping: Here's a little play on words when it comes to mushrooms. Have you heard about rage rooms? These are places where you can go and suit up in protective gear, choose a weapon, and then enter a room and smash everything for a prepaid time to release rage. Hmm, sounds interesting but also expensive and exhausting. So skip the rage room and try a session with rage shrooms! Chop them, break them in half with your hands, whatever it takes to make you feel better and release pent-up energy, stress, or anger.

Cooking: Next, cook the mushrooms in the style of your choosing. Whether you pan sear or roast, mushrooms release water and mirror a "reduction," ending up a little flatter but with all the flavor intact. Observe how they change and think about releasing what's holding you back from being at your best. What stress and anger can you release from your life to promote well-being for yourself and the other "mushrooms" in your life?

Squash

There are so many different types of squash and so many ways to feel bad about ourselves. Could there be a better semantic metaphor for ridding yourself of negativity and low self-esteem? Here is a little primer for reversing negative self-talk with a few different kinds of squash:

Butternut Squash

Precut squash: One way to be easy on yourself is to resolve to buy butternut squash already cubed! As you prepare it, you will be so happy to remove the arduous steps of halving it safely and scooping out the mess. Now marry this ease with being easy on yourself.

Cooking: Pick one negative self-talk comment you tell yourself or worry loop that's come to roost in your mind and imagine it shrinking and softening as the cubes will. No matter how you cook it, butternut squash softens, and so can you.

Acorn Squash

Cooking: Pop a full squash in the microwave for a minute or two and think about how quickly and intensely that appliance changes squash from hard to soft. Now you can halve it more easily.

If you'll do it for squash, why not for yourself? If something has been hard to accomplish, ask yourself if you've really given your all, intensely and with commitment, like that microwave. Additionally, perhaps you can soften just one way you've been acting or thinking and watch how easy it becomes to look inside yourself. Once you learn and practice the skill of taking a moment or two to "cut in," it will help exponentially and you will always be able to "see" what's going on inside.

Summer Squash

Slicing or chopping: Whether it's green or yellow, summer squash is delicious with the peel. Though we do peel off in a lot of recipes, this time let's talk about keeping the peel on to recognize and seal in what's working. Sometimes we focus too much on flaws, whereas recognizing strengths could be more impactful than working on perceived problems. Slice or chop your squash, but don't think about reducing it; think about how all of the pieces combine for something delicious, and if possible use both green and yellow. Notice the color combination and name something bright and beautiful about yourself. Then think about what's below your peel that's a strength or a positive trait and say it out loud. Let it live in the air and in your head and heart for a full minute before you proceed. When we tangibly identify our strengths, they stick longer.

Root vegetables (potatoes, carrots, radishes, beets, and turnips)

Could there be a better metaphor for getting to the root of what's bothering us or holding us back? Is it a behavior, a feeling, a communication style, or negative self-talk? When you use a root vegetable, first take a mindful moment to try to define a nebulous feeling more clearly or shine a light on a pattern that's been buried "deep in the ground," aka inside yourself, but that you know is not working. Root vegetables have to be pulled out, and sometimes you have to tug hard because they're deeply implanted, just like habitual methods of communicating or behaving. If you've told yourself anything negative about yourself, pull it out now and peel or chop or boil it away. If you recognize something you do that's not been working, vow to try a different method as you add these to your dish. Breaking habits is hard, but the only way to do it is to highlight it, then try something new.

Dairy

Milk (cow's, almond, oat, low-fat, dairy-free, coconut)

Pouring: Are you pouring milk into a cake or shake? Adding it to a sauce? Depending on how you use it, there are similarities and differences. When we pour any substance, we can think about either pouring in positives, like resolve or strength or gratitude, or pouring away negatives, such as unhappiness, grief, or negative self-talk. The coolness of milk gives us the opportunity to do both.

Think about what's firing hot in your life that needs to cool down, like a relationship or work or financial situation or even your own worry or anger. Then use milk as a tangible representation of pouring coolness into the mix to settle things down.

Adding small amounts: If you're simply adding a tablespoon or two into a sauce, try to think of one or two small acts of kindness you can do for yourself or others, or name one or two things that are going well in your life. Therapy shouldn't be just problem focused. Recognizing what's working is important too, as that can be an area to mine for future action. It should be used as a tool and blueprint for going forward when a challenge arises. Additionally, highlighting what's worked in the past and what you've done well is a boost to self-esteem.

Yogurt

What is yogurt? Even though I eat yogurt almost every day, I can't help thinking of it as a bacteria that has fermented, and if it were described that way on the package, it's likely that none of us would be eating it. Guess what? That's a great way of thinking about ourselves. How are we describing ourselves to the world? And how are we thinking about ourselves to, you guessed it, ourselves? How we feel about who we are can be changed if need be, just the way yogurt changes. When you spoon or open yogurt, ask yourself *Am I focusing on my perceived flaws, some that I may have "let ferment" for years, and letting that define me, or can I accept that while I may have "bacteria," I may also come together as someone smooth and cool and creamy and wonderful, full of different flavors?* Did you know that before the fermentation process in yogurt, it's also full of sugars?

To recap, when you use yogurt, think about acceptance, letting go of secrets that aren't working for you, and remembering to always name a few of your "sugars" out loud.

Butter/Ghee

Years ago, I was invited to a farm in upstate New York to milk goats. It was messy, but I did see the staff turn the goat milk into all kinds of products, including butter. I never forgot the idea of transformation and how something so raw and messy could be turned into so many delicious things.

Softening or melting: Butter is a great tool for an emotional makeover. It's often cold and hard, and to be used, it needs to be either softened or melted. The next time you're spreading butter or melting it in a glass or pan, think about converting one or two "pats" (traits) that may currently be hard or cold in your life. Bring them to room temperature. You do have the power to take a mess and turn it around.

If using ghee, then it's all about separating the solids and ending up with something clear. Think about that for yourself. Is there a big chunk of solid thought process that's been with you forever and weighing you down, keeping you from a new way of thinking or acting?

When you melt butter or ghee, you may also want to think about any time you've had a meltdown. We all have them, but it's a good time to remind yourself that while melting down is helpful in a recipe, it's probably much less so in life.

Add more butter! I also like the idea of making life a little more buttery. Too often our busy lives are moving quickly, and with stress and little time, we forget to just be, with our families or ourselves. Just be cozy and buttery.

Cheese (all types)

Layering: If you are layering a slice on a sandwich, then we need to talk about layers, and cheese is often a representation of what we want in life, tangibly, such as money, fame, success, and possessions as well as a relationship and/or family. I'm going to ask you to layer differently. If you're only adding one slice, take a mindful moment and name one thing that's working in your life or in your personality—like an affirmation. Take a moment and layer in something optimistic, like "I'm going to remember to smile and laugh more each day," and let it stick.

There's power in tangible positivity; it has legs to make all the other things happen. When we say things like "I wish I had more money," it doesn't stick the same way. Unlike the cheese, which generally stays put, wishing without a plan for material things is more like the lettuce in a sandwich that can fall off or move around.

Sprinkle, shred, or grate: The other way you may be using cheese is to sprinkle it, perhaps shredded or grated. If anything is making you feel shredded, any situation or person, or if you're doing it to yourself with negative self-talk, here is an opportunity to have a strong experiential moment and pull those feelings out of you and send them on their way. In other words, excavate them from inside you and give them to the cheese. Then, as you sprinkle or add shredded cheese to a dish, take those devaluing feelings and add them to the dish. If it happens to be a dish where the cheese melts, even better; say goodbye to it as it melts. If the cheese is in a dish such as a salad, that's fine; toss all the other ingredients around it and make those negative traits less prominent, less dominating. Obviously, one act such as this doesn't turn everything around, but it's a start and a powerful thought to take with you. Like cheese, toxic situations or people that have too much "air" begin to get moldy and smell. It's the same with giving them airtime in your head or gut. Toxic thoughts will make you feel as rotten as cheese gone bad.

That's why sprinkling is a perfect metaphor for unloading negative people or situations. It's a visual act of saying goodbye and resolving to move forward with freshness.

Grated cheese is almost always sprinkled, one of my favorite cooking therapy acts. Usually we sprinkle grated cheese on top of things. It's a nice time to think about whether you're on top of your plans, wishes, and pursuits and, if not, a reminder to focus or refocus on your dreams or goals. If you've been detoured, it might be internally "grating" like the cheese, and this metaphor can be both a reminder of what you want and a strategy to recognize and sprinkle away some of the sharp and annoying sounds of whatever's grating you. Years ago, my grandmother would grate things by hand on an old-fashioned grater that would always cut her, and she'd say, "A little bit of blood is okay; it's the love in the dish." Yikes. I loved my grandma, but I do disagree. There's absolutely no reason to keep grating and bleeding into your life. Sprinkle away anything cutting and move forward.

Spreading: Most spreadable cheeses like goat cheese or burrata or cream cheese lend themselves perfectly to adding aspirations. Spreading cheese is an act of hope and a perfect time to think about dreams and goals. Whether you're spreading it onto bread, crackers, or veggies, name three things you'd like to add to your life as you do. Once again, these are realistic but can be far reaching. For instance, you can say that you'd like to be able to afford a new house one day. Spread that in. You can hope to meet someone who will become a lifelong partner. Spread that in. You can even state that you'd like to get your dream job or dream vacation. Tangibly stating a goal makes it more likely to happen, as it cements intent.

Whipped Cream (homemade, canned, or in a tub)

Texture and temperature: Whether you are making it yourself, spraying it out of a can, or scooping from a tub, whipped cream is going to be cool and creamy. It is usually added to a dish and is not the main dish. So, either way you're using it, think about something you've been adding to your life, whether at work, at home, or internally, that brings down pain or sadness or tension, like a colleague you can share with or a hobby that's fulfilling or a decision to be more at peace with yourself. Take a mindful moment to spell it out and let it take shape. Just as the whipped cream has gone from liquid to semisolid, let your thoughts do the same. That's another metaphor: Whipped cream takes work, whether being pressurized in a can or whipped in a bowl. Are you the only one charged with keeping things cool? The only one doing the work? That may be just fine with you, but this is a more layered ingredient than you might have thought, even though it's a topping. It's great to inject coolness, associated with calm, but it's not great to be the only one doing it. If that's the case, take a moment to recognize it and decide how you want to "top things off" going forward.

Squirting from a can: The can is pressurized. As you spray or squirt, it's an excellent time to let some of the pressure out that you may have in your life, as we all do at times. When you do it consciously, even just that squirt with your thumb in charge can be a powerful cooking therapy process.

Whipping by hand: If you are whipping your own cream, then you know that it must be watched carefully for just the right amount of time. Is any person or situation in your life requiring that sort of attention? Some moments in life are demanding in an expected way. Little children need watching. Work requires diligence. Partners have needs. But take this moment to determine if anyone or anything is taking up too much of your time. Think about the noise of it as you whip. Perhaps all is well and this noise is not irritating or loud but just in the background or even calming, and that's great. But if not, what could you do a little differently to turn down the noise of being in demand? Either way, consciously decide.

Scooping from a tub: When we scoop something cool and creamy out of a tub, it's a chance to take a mindful moment and notice the fluffiness and softness. No matter what we're going through, all of us have memories of soft and fluffy times or moments in our lives. When we add this to a bowl of pudding or ice cream, it's a time to name one or two things that are working in our lives or have worked in the past. As I've said before, naming things we've achieved or accomplished reminds us of successes, provides a sense of mastery, and not only improves our self-outlook but is actually incredibly effective for problem-solving as we go forward.

Ice Cream/Frozen Yogurt/Gelato

If you've ever made your own ice cream or any frozen dessert, you know that frozen desserts freeze slowly, over time. This is reminiscent of annoyances, displeasures, and pet peeves. We may accept behaviors or habits or even mindsets that are irritating or uncomfortable to be nice or compliant or compromise. Many minor irritations never get to the point where we are internally icy over those behaviors and the need to tolerate them. But if there are things you've been allowing to slowly freeze or things that are already frozen in your life and they are keeping you hard-hearted instead of soft, and you've even tried to "let them sit and soften" but with no luck, you may now need to scoop them out as you scoop your ice cream into the bowl. This can be a relationship with a toxic partner or friend, an extended family relationship that is always negative, a work situation where you are devalued and frustrated, or even a sense that you've lost yourself in your own life. If we continue with the ice cream metaphor, perhaps you've always loved chocolate but are stuck in a strawberry life. This may be a time to think about being your own flavor, the one you were meant to be. Again, we don't make big changes from one cooking therapy session, but we do think about them.

Protein

Beans

Though used regularly in many cultural cuisines, beans are often a "sneaky" way to get protein in a meal. Whether or not that's your intent, I like to think about three possibilities when it comes to using beans and the metaphor of sneaking in: First, ask yourself whether anything has been slowly or surreptitiously bothering you and whether, instead of addressing it, if you've been letting it go or even grow. Have you heard of sneaker waves? These are waves that come in without warning at the beach. You never know when they're going to happen, but suddenly after minutes or even hours of manageable waves, a sneaker wave comes in that is higher and stronger and can be unexpectedly harmful. Secrets and frustrations that build can be like sneaker waves. Ask yourself if you've been keeping any secrets that have been sneakily starting to interfere with your personal peace or outlook.

If so, soak the beans to soften them, and use this as a mindful moment to think about your next steps. A more positive metaphor for beans being sneaky is to think about what you can easily sneak into your day as a positive or healthy act for you or someone else. Resolve to take a walk or embrace nature in any way you choose. Check on an elderly or sick neighbor or relative. Put down the phone in a doctor's office and have a conversation instead.

Chicken (uncooked)

To wash or not to wash? There is some debate over whether to wash raw chicken and whether or not that act can spread the potential for bacteria or lessen it, but the FDA recommends washing chicken, and so you should. But as you proceed, this is a moment to think about the way you interact with everyone in your life. Do you do whatever you can so as not to spread emotional bacteria? Are you gentle and kind with the people in your life, conscious of their feelings and never passive-aggressive, and do you receive the same in return? In this way, just from a discussion of handling the chicken, we have our first opportunity to think about how we are being treated and how we treat others. You don't have to act, just take a mindful moment to recognize.

Preparing to cook: With raw chicken it's important to pay attention to semantics. Whether you are going to bake, roast, fry, or sauté, the chicken starts out raw. Yes, you want to think about anything that's making you feel raw or undone, that's important to identify. But also, try to remember a time when you were still learning and absorbing, a time when you were fresh and raw, in a good way, before situations and attitudes and lifestyles were "cooked" into you. Do you need to go back to that time in your memory and examine whether you've absorbed as much of the promises and plans for yourself that you wanted to or can? Just handling that slippery raw chicken can give you a chance to see what slipped away, or better yet, what you can slip in now.

No matter how you're going to prepare raw chicken, think about changing something raw into something eatable. Yes, *eatable* is another semantic metaphor. We often use the word *delicious* to describe a person or experience, and the word *eatable* is at the root of that adjective. Have you ever looked at a baby and said they were so adorable you could "eat them up"? Think about whether you're eatable, aspiring to be, or insisting that others in your life aspire to the same standard. Raw chicken, and people, can make you sick. As you turn the oven or stove on to cook your chicken, resolve to "heat up" your intention to have more deliciousness in your life.

Chicken (cooked)

Removing the skin: I love the metaphor of removing the skin to see what's underneath. If we're not used to therapy or self-examination, it can be that we've been covered in a familiar, unchanging skin of habits and patterns. Removing the skin is a commitment to look at ourselves in a different way.

Pulling apart: Rotisserie chicken, or chicken on the bone, can be pulled, which is wonderful for taking a moment to think about what may be pulling us in a wrong direction, or even what's been pulling us apart. Naming any of these things is the first step to changing them.

Chopping or shredding: Whether you are using your chicken in a salad or casserole, you may also need to chop it into smaller pieces. As you do so, use the chopping as a metaphor for breaking down any unclear negative feelings into recognizable items you can address. For example, as you chop "anger," change it into a piece of one thing that makes you angry. If you chop "boredom," then name exactly what is boring and maybe even one small piece that might make a difference. Finally, add your chopped pieces of actual, named things to the dish and sit with this new knowledge. You can either think about change if you're heating, or if you're having a salad or sandwich, let it sit cold. Either way, you should now have a more focused idea of what you want.

Ground meat (beef, chicken, turkey, lamb, or pork)

Changing shape: Whether you are making patties, meatballs, meatloaf, or taco meat, when it comes to ground meat, there will be some sort of shaping or changing of state. Since there are so many ways to use this ingredient, let's concentrate on going from an unrecognizable lump to something that looks like a dish you'd like to prepare. If you're searching, figuring out next steps, simply contemplating where you are, or even acknowledging that you're totally lost, getting your hands in the mix is a great metaphor for taking control. Let's face it, meat is not the sexiest ingredient, but it can stand for strength or brawn and getting to "the meat of the matter." So shape it into balls, sculpt it into a loaf, pound it into patties, and think about taking control of something. Even if you are in a good place, there's always room to think about the next steps.

When I lost my mom, I decided to evaluate what I could do to live my best life to honor her, and I vowed three things: Do a job I love, laugh more with my children, love more with my spouse. The point is, shape the meat and think about sculpting something that's misshapen, rough, or jagged into a rounded or better "state", or if all is on running smoothly, shape the next step.

Salmon (or the fish of your choice)

Trusting your gut: When you prepare salmon or any fish, you often sniff it to make sure it doesn't smell too "fishy." I love that metaphor for trusting your gut! Does anything feel "fishy" in your life right now? Instead of ignoring those warning bells, trust your intuition. I once heard that the worst lie you can tell is the lie you tell yourself. Think about that as the salmon sizzles or bakes.

Salmon or other skin: And if you're making salmon with the skin on, make sure you like the skin you're in as well.

Flaky texture: Finally, when cooked right, salmon should be flaky. Guess what? I love a little flaky in my life, and I believe so should we all. By flaky, I mean it's okay to have our quirks and idiosyncrasies that add individuality, dimension, and even whimsy to ourselves. As we grow, we also sometimes loose our silliness and playfulness, and as you cut into your salmon, please think about how you can "cut in" some healthy playtime to your life.

Eggs

Cracking the egg: I think eggs may have been put on this earth to be an ingredient in cooking therapy. One of the first times I worked with a client and we cracked eggs, I asked her to think of a metaphor for the act, and she blurted out, "It's me! I'm cracked!" Oh boy, now that was a challenge to dispel. We spent most of the session building up her self-concept and "filling" her with the other ingredients. If you are feeling like you're in pieces, please feel free to crack the eggs and embrace that feeling, but also laugh a little at the image and "crack yourself up"? Then, as the egg pours out, have a mindful moment and think about the yolk, about how it represents new life and how you can consider the same. Throw away the old "shell" (yes, that's you right now) and let the idea of change and possibility live in whatever dish you are making with eggs. This is not the time to "walk on eggshells" with yourself.

    Boiling: If you are not cracking your egg because you are making soft or hard-boiled eggs, imagine yourself as solid and contained and powerful. When you eventually peel away the shell, you can peel away any negative emotions that may be holding you back from that power. I always plunge my newly hard-boiled eggs into ice water for five to ten minutes, because then the shell will peel right off. I suspect if you take down your negative self-talk or communication style that isn't working, the same will happen for you. Rather than engaging in a hard, tedious task, you can slide *your* sharp, uneatable shell off more easily than you ever imagined.

Scrambling: Cracking eggs open is an equally powerful way to have a cooking therapy session. As you crack the egg open and pour it into a bowl, imagine that you're opening yourself up and that you're pouring something that's been bothering you into the bowl. In other words, you're removing it from yourself and putting it out there where it can be changed. You can choose a personality trait, such as "I'm always impatient." Or you might state a challenge that you're having, such as "I'm overwhelmed at work," or it can be something you'd like to change, such as "I have to make more time for myself." Take a mindful moment before you do anything else and say out loud this one thing.

As you whisk the eggs to combine them, take your one trait and think of a possible solution. For example, if you're impatient, you might plan to add meditation to your day. If it's a work situation, perhaps you'll decide to speak to your supervisor. If you need more personal time, you may need to examine time management. Once you have a solution in your mind, imagine adding it to the problem in the bowl and whisking away the problem with the solution. Now you have only a mixture of solutions, because you've made a plan to address the problems. Pour the "remedy" into your hot pan and imagine the resolution being "cooked in." Whether you mix it up for scrambled eggs or allow it to solidify for an omelet, your eggs will be brightly colored and firm and your plan will be equally solid.

Quinoa/Buckwheat

Unlike some plant proteins, quinoa and buckwheat are complete proteins, meaning they contain all nine essential amino acids that our bodies cannot make on their own.

Proteins are made up of amino acids strung together in a chain. Think about the quinoa or buckwheat as a template of you; a chain of traits, habits, and actions you can string together for change, self-improvement, or calm.

Naturally, I'd like you to take a moment and think about your own image and whether you're projecting who you really are to the world but also to yourself. In other words, do you look like rice, a starch (and starchy), when you are really quinoa, packed with a protein punch that no one has seen? If you want to change, first you need to identify who you are and begin to think about who you'd like to be and what you'd like to change or add to get there. Identification is the first step. These changes aren't necessarily huge, like altering a career or lifestyle. They can be small, such as adding a hobby or getting outside more or smiling at strangers as you pass by.

Soaking up water: Your quinoa or buckwheat may cook a little differently, but both will need to soak up water as they cook. Before you pour the water into the pot, imagine filling it with anything you'd like to add to your life. This could be tangible, like hydrating more, or a personality trait, such as being more tolerant or courageous. It's your decision. This ingredient represents you, and it is going to soak up what you put into it.

Seasoning: When it's ready, you may add spices or seasoning. Take a mindful moment to reflect on what you've put into the dish and any changes you'll make going forward.

Deli Meats

Even if you're just putting together a sandwich, there's so much to gain from cooking therapy.

Layering: Usually deli meats are in slices, which is a great metaphor for layering or layers in your life. Years ago, I was involved in a project called Green Circle, which encouraged participants to create a circle with the center being their most important people or tasks and each outer circle being progressively filled with less important people or obligations. It was a great visual for prioritizing.

As you layer your slices, create your own Green Circle. You will likely begin with some sort of bread, which is your outer layer. In this session, bread represents minor pursuits or "actors" in your life. It may be a neighbor or a museum you visit once a month or even a medical condition you must watch. Next, perhaps lettuce? You're getting closer to the "meat" but not there yet. Perhaps this represents extended family, a task you do weekly at home or work, or a hobby that keeps you feeling fresh. If you are adding things like tomato or onion, keep thinking about getting closer to the people and things that are important to you, and when you add the deli meat and close the sandwich, you will have created a tangible reminder of what's important.

Here is an alternate way to do this short session. Each layer represents a part of your personality that is positive. This is a session on applause. Often we give so much airtime in our heads to flaws and mistakes and so little to our actual achievements and successes. Each time you layer a slice, say out loud one thing that's great about you. It can be a tangible achievement, like doing a great job at work, or you can transform a personality trait into a tangible achievement, like "I always add goodness to myself and others." Keep layering and adding positive self-talk. That sandwich will close and be the most delicious you've ever had!

Pasta

For All Types

Boiling: Remind yourself that softening is always a good strategy for good communication, happy relationships, and creating calm.

If there is something going on that is "boiling and bubbling" and does need your attention, now is the time to turn up the heat on the water in the pot. Think of heat as a catalyst for change, both literally and figuratively, and if you've been being boiling mad, bring those mad bubbles of discontent to the surface.

Add the noodles slowly, because we never want to add the pasta all at once, right? Take a similar approach with any problems you have; don't overwhelm yourself with a mountain of woes. Try to think about crystallizing one or two things that are "hard" for you right now and contributing to anger or frustration. You don't have to try to fix them yet or make them "softer." Just identify. There'll be time enough later to "mix solutions" into the sauce. Don't add a whole pound in, or the clumps of noodles will stick together, just like the problems, and they'll stay hard and difficult to digest. Then be mindful of gently stirring to loosen the pasta and yourself. This is your work for now.

Once you've softened the pasta and cooked in one or two issues instead of a boiling mass, you will eventually "turn off" the heat and the water will cool down. Now you can decide on a few things to work on and refer to the session recipes in each section to create a session for yourself and add potential solutions. Chapter 6 even has a session with pasta, called "Feeling Brand Newdles," for creating calm.

Long Noodles (angel hair, linguine, spaghetti, etc.)

Long noodles give us a chance to take a "long" look at softening and hardening. But first, before you place the pasta in the boiling water, take note of its length and make a mindful decision to take that long look at yourself. When your water is ready and boiling, slowly add your pasta to the water and think about how when you submerge the noodles in water, the first parts of the pasta will soften, and then you will gently push the second parts in and stir.

Think about yourself. What have you submerged in terms of hard and soft parts of yourself? Are there parts of you that need to soften? Or parts of you that are too soft? Have you been too hard on yourself or others? Or too "mushy" liked overcooked pasta? Think about your relationships and your communication style. What could benefit from a softer or tougher consistency? As the pasta boils, try to imagine creating a balance that is more "al dente," just soft and just firm enough.

Breaking in half: If you are someone who likes to break long noodles like angel hair, linguine, or spaghetti in half, listen for that little crack when you break them. Think about cracking yourself open so that you can explore things going on inside. Is anything broken? Does anything need a little glue or to be repaired?

Short Noodles (penne, cavatappi, rigatoni, macaroni shells, elbow, etc.)

Shapes: Short noodles come in so many different shapes, just like people, personalities, moods, and degrees of emotional balance. Let's do a little check on your homeostasis by looking at some of the many shapes of these pastas. If you're using rigatoni, which has lines, ask yourself to measure the lines of communication you have going on with family, friends, and colleagues. Do it purposefully and honestly. Shells? Think about your outer shell. Hard, like the pasta is now, or soft enough to soak up warmth from the hot water? Elbows? Let's use the semantic metaphor and focus on whether you're putting elbow grease or enough work into creating opportunities for the things you enjoy and/or the people you love. Spirals? This is a chance to think deeply about your direction in terms of your own happiness and satisfaction. Are you spiraling up in terms of getting what you want? Or have you been on a downward spiral in terms of self-care and attaining your goals? Take a hard look at where you are and where you'd like to be.

Rice (long grain, short grain, arborio, etc.)

If you've read the section on quinoa, you know that I love to use ingredients that "absorb," and so it is with rice. Whether it's long grain, short grain, or arborio, all rice is going to give you the little gift of forty minutes or so to contemplate. Now some of you may think of that gift as a curse because you've never sat with yourself or your thoughts for that long perhaps ever, and I understand that. But this ingredient can take some of your dissatisfactions from "grainy" to "wholly clear." Are you with me? If so, choose your liquid. I like to use vegetable or chicken stock instead of water because it's more flavorful, and that's a perfect metaphor for taking stock of what's coming together and what you're absorbing. The best definition of happiness I've heard describes it as "something to do, someone to love, something to hope for." So instead of asking if you're happy, ask yourself, "Am I doing work that fulfills me?" Ask, "Do I have enough love and support for me?" And "Do I feel content and at peace?" These are better measures for a "happy" life. These are the goals to absorb as the rice cooks. When all the liquid is absorbed, remove the rice from the pot and take a mindful moment to think about all of the grains as aspirations as well as accomplishments and characteristics you've achieved.

Baking Items

Flour (all types: sifted, unsifted, gluten-free, almond, oat)

A baking base: No matter the flour you use, I always think of it as the staff of life. Flour is the base for so many dishes and can hold everything together. For that reason, imagine the flour as you, as your base, for all your choices and personality traits and actions to come. When you add it, no matter the measure, think about it being a kind of blank slate. Flour can remind you that you are an individual with free will and you can still make new choices and add or subtract who you are today, depending on what's working for you.

    Sifting: As you sift flour, think similarly about removing any "hard rocks or pieces" that ruin the dish. Think about what's left when you sift through your life, your relationships, your feelings and behaviors, with an open eye toward becoming a smoother, powderier you. When you eventually add the flour to the dish, think about how it will add substance to whatever you're making; even if it's just a slurry for a sauce, the flour can hold things together. With some self-examination, I'm sure you too can get or keep it all together.

Be silly: Have a little fun with flour. Put some on your hands and clap them together. Yes, I know it creates a little mess, but that should never stop us from channeling the silly little kid inside. I try to bring mine out at least once a day, because smiles and sillies reaps heaps of emotional benefits.

Sugar (or sugar substitutes like stevia, Splenda, Truvia, Equal, Sweet'n Low, monkfruit)

Love and kindness: The obvious metaphor for using sugar is to think about all of the sweetness that exists in your life, but let's also think about people or places in your life that could benefit from your kindness. Why talk about where sugar could improve others? It has to do with giving. I think we can go deeper when using sugar. Charitable acts have been shown to add benefits equally to the giver and recipient.

In the Resources section at the end of this book, you can read about a study at the Cleveland Clinic, which shows that a chemical reaction takes place in your body from doing something nice and causes your brain to activate all of the "feel-good" chemicals like dopamine, serotonin, and oxytocin. Believe it or not, being charitable contributes to lower blood pressure and—wait for it—blood *sugar*. How perfect is that?

So yes, sprinkle or add sugar and think about the sweetness in your life. As I always say, we don't focus enough on what's going well and tend to ruminate on what we perceive isn't. But also, think of one place where you can make a difference. You don't have to join an organization or make a large donation; perhaps just make a phone call or visit to an elderly neighbor or relative. You decide, in your own "sweet time."

Baking Powder and Soda

We've all heard the expression "packs a punch" to describe small things that have large impact, like a spicy chili pepper or a dollop of wasabi or even an alcoholic drink that is very strong. Well, these small-dose ingredients just may pack the punchiest, and my most favorite, metaphor, "Help rise." Do you hear choir bells ringing? I do. Helping yourself to rise is at the core of self-talk. When we think about creating or changing a habit, self-talk is number one on my list. We know that baking powder and soda don't add taste to a batter. Rather, they help the bread (or brownies or cake), rise.

Here is your assignment just before you add either or both of these ingredients: Stop for a moment, step back, and physically stretch your body tall, throw your shoulders back, stand on your tiptoes if you can, and raise your arms in the air high above your head. Reach for the sky and rise up. This small movement can set the tone for the rest of your day. Notice how it feels to get out of your head for a moment and into your body, and think about this act as a metaphor for rising up in whatever part of your life you choose. When you add the teaspoon or half teaspoon of powder or soda, think about how a little change in belief can change what you tell yourself and impact your thoughts and behaviors in a big way. Rise up in your head to rise up in your life.

Vanilla

Stirring in: Through the years vanilla has been used aromatically, medicinally, and even to treat skin conditions. I like the idea that one little teaspoon of a substance can be so utilitarian, which is why when I use vanilla in a cooking therapy session. I ask the client to imprint the vanilla with their own aspirations. That means to imagine that the vanilla represents anything you want or dream about, from something tangible like a new job to an emotional pursuit such as courage. It's a chance to put it out there into the universe. Take a moment and think about it mindfully and purposely. Consider it a liquid dream board if that resonates. It's impossible to attain something if we don't first identify and own it.

Cinnamon (nutmeg, allspice, ginger, cloves)

Mixing: You can't eat cinnamon alone because it's far too bitter. It's the same with any of the spices you may choose. They are sweet when mixed with the right ingredients. I think this is a great metaphor for cementing relationships you already have, letting others into your life, and asking for help when you need it. It can be hard to ask people for help, and many clients I've worked with feel a fair amount of failure and shame when they do. But people need people! And we often forget how good it feels when someone asks for our help or advice. Rather than alienating someone when you ask for help, it can create a bond. In fact, studies have shown that loneliness can shorten a person's life span by fifteen years. How can you become more social or more involved in your community? In what areas of your life can you ask for help? If you're struggling with any type of mental health issue or disorder, find someone safe to talk to and with whom you can honestly share. Think about community, concerns, and connection with cinnamon (they all begin with a C!). Seek out companionship with a capital C and solidifying the positive relationships you already have.

Salt

Let's talk about some of the idioms for salt and how every time you add it to a recipe, you can customize it to what suits you at that time.

- *Don't pour salt in the wound* instructs one not to make a bad situation worse. Before you add salt to a dish, take a mental step back and think about that before you physically do it. Think about a situation that's upsetting. Take a pause.
- *"Take it with a grain of salt."* You know, I believe a healthy dose of doubt is often a good thing. Whether it's a financial deal or a piece of gossip, a step back is always a good thing. Before you add the salt, if something in your life feels sketchy or too good to be true, take it slow. However, if someone has given you a compliment, feel free to take it with a heaping dose of *no* salt!

- *Salt of the earth.* This phrase dates back to the New Testament and describes someone who is honest and reliable. The older I get, the more I want the people in my life to mirror this phrase and have these attributes and the more I try to be that for them. I hope you have loving friends in your life who are "the salt of the earth," and if not, try to find them. I often say that I learn from my clients in session, and this is one of those really important moments that always reminds both Sherpa and climber to review and reflect. As you add the salt, think about who is "adding" to your life and who is just a little "too salty."

- *Back to the salt mines.* If you happen to be in a rut, experiencing malaise, or perhaps in a role or two that feels like drudgery, adding salt at this moment can represent those feelings and bring them out into the light. Adding salt is adding flavor. Perhaps it's time to wake up some old dreams that have taken a back seat to responsibility or at least explore a hobby that can add flavor. If this feels like you, then salt is a prompt to make a change. You can't even begin to make a change until you know what's "down in the salt mines" and name it. Try to purposefully say out loud that you commit to addressing ways to add flavor to your life, relationship, or situation.

Nuts (walnuts, peanuts, cashews, pistachios, pinenuts, pecans)

Go nuts! There are times in life when there is just no other choice than to go nuts. If you can add nuts to every meal just so you can "go nuts," I highly recommend it. You've heard me say often that many of us have lost the "silly" in our lives. That's such a shame. Add nuts and go nuts. Do a little happy dance right in the middle of your kitchen.

Versatility: By the way, did you ever realize that nuts go well with almost anything? Think about it: meat dishes, veggies, breakfasts, desserts? Maybe it's because we're supposed to add a little frivolity to our lives every day. I'm a big fan of whimsy and fun and healthy spontaneity. Studies show that occasional silliness can reduce tension and stress.

Dried Spices and Herbs

Salt and Pepper

Although we've already covered salt extensively, I wanted to address salt and pepper together because they are so frequently a part of recipes and often we are asked to "salt and pepper to taste." If you notice, the phrase "salt and pepper to taste" acts like a noun and a verb; it's both a substance and an action, and I believe that can be a blueprint for life. Our lives are the substance, and we continually try to live in a way where we feel balanced and flavored "just right." This is a work in progress, the verb of the process. We add and subtract, continually trying to get it "just right." With salt and pepper, we're creating a balance, and we add them to a recipe not necessarily in equal parts, but together. Adding balance to life is exactly the same; we have so many parts and need to remember to examine the amounts and adjust accordingly. As you add salt and pepper to your dish, this is a great time to think about where you may need to adjust, if at all, what you're putting into the various "dishes" of your life. Family, work, leisure, and emotional health can all get "out of balance." Checking in is key and salt and pepper can be an excellent reminder to do so.

Garlic

We know that a head of garlic has many cloves or parts. Is this possibly a time to make room for developing some of your other parts? They say that no matter how many children a parent has, for example, they can keep growing chambers in their heart to love each one. I think it's the same for people in general. Don't limit yourself with finite talk about who you are; think of ways to grow exponentially, and you will be more interesting to others and yourself and open up opportunities for joy.

Vibrant Spices (paprika, chili powder, pumpkin spice)

These spices are brightly colored, primarily reds and oranges, and I call them the "vibrants." When you add a spice with color, it's a great time to think about whether you're living life in color or black and white—and by this I mean not just going through the motions. There is a phrase in therapy that asks *Are you living life or is life living you?* This means are you merely a vessel for other people's plans and allowing circumstances to dictate what you do, where you live or work, and who you're with? Or are you doing things purposefully, making choices based on your needs and desires? It's an important question. Over time, if you're not advocating for yourself, you risk becoming dissatisfied and resentful.

When we add any of the colorful spices to dishes, it's to add intense color, flavor, and brightness. If we leave these spices out, the dish suffers. It's an easy leap to imagine what happens if we are doing the same with our lives. Why serve up a lesser flavor of ourselves? Every time you add a colorful spice, remind yourself to seek zest. Even with intense responsibilities or structure, there is always room to add a hint or pinch of passion.

Fresh Herbs (oregano, basil, parsley)

I call these green herbs the "freshies." Anytime I add an ingredient that is green or leafy to a dish, I think of fresh starts, newness, and nature. Adding these herbs is a clarion call to remember your inner Zen and humanity. Ask yourself *Have I been taking care of myself physically and emotionally? Am I nourishing my soul as well as my body? What more can I do to replace any staleness that has crept in with inspiration and spirit?*

Sprinkling herbs into a dish to add freshness makes me think of random acts of kindness. As you add any of these "freshies," think about one thing you can do for someone else as well as yourself.

Whole Seeds (fennel, sesame, poppy)

Even if you decide to crush or grind whole seeds, when you start with them, you are "planting." Ask yourself whether any new ideas, decisions, or changes need to be planted. This is a chance to examine what is already firmly planted in terms of your lifestyle or mindset and whether or not it's working.

Alternately, is it possible that something is too firmly planted and could benefit from a little loosening, a little diluting with water, or a little freshening with sunlight? Even more, perhaps your mindset is not firm enough and a little too loosely planted. If so, chances are it won't "set." Additionally, who is doing the planting? If someone else is deciding what needs to be done and when, then you've lost control of your own growth. Once again, as you add seeds, analyze what needs to grow and what needs to be weeded out.

Aromatic Spices (cumin, turmeric, cardamom, saffron)

These spices are aromatic and add a special quality to a dish. So when you use these spices, the idea is to think about adding a little glamour or allure to your life. I don't care if you live on a farm or a mountaintop or a riverboat; all of us need to feel beautiful and fascinating at times. It may seem superficial, especially if you're not used to a sparkly scarf or aromatic perfume or cologne, but push yourself out of that comfort zone just to see how you feel when you add something snazzy, especially if you're not used to doing that. There is so much to explore in the world and so much benefit in newness. And it doesn't have to be a tangible good. You can take a class or dance by yourself or have an adventurous drive or trip. Add the aromatic spices and plan to add pizazz.

Kitchen Staples

Oil (olive, coconut, canola, avocado, grapeseed, vegetable, infused)

Holding together: Whether you're adding oil to a batter, a marinade, or a pan, it's going to do a job. It's not so much a flavor as it is a *reason*. Oil is going to thicken or coat or seep or hold other ingredients together. When using oil, it's a time to think about how you're doing and how you're holding it all together. Maybe it's an opportunity to examine all the parts of you and your situation or maybe just a chance to self-applaud. Oil can "break apart" or "separate." If that's not happening and you're doing it all and it's working, then you may be the "grease that holds it all together." If so, then as you add the oil, give yourself some kudos and enjoy the pour.

Vinegar (white wine, red wine, white, rice wine, champagne, apple cider, balsamic, infused)

No matter the type of vinegar, there will be some acidity. Let's take a hard look at ourselves and ask what sorts of vibes we're putting into the world. All of us default to our smallest selves at times, becoming jealous or gossipy or simply lashing out at a loved one for a reason other than the one we may express. Acidity in vinegar will balance a dish. Acidity in tone, words, or feelings will do the opposite for you. This is not to be self-scolding but rather for us to hold ourselves to a higher and kinder standard each and every day. It's circuitous; not only do we improve the lives of others but also ourselves. We can consciously make a choice to be softer and kinder. Begin with an hour, a day, and turn a new practice into a habit. Additionally, do not accept a constant barrage of acidic remarks or treatment from others. Also, you may have heard the phrase to describe someone who is bold and confident as "full of spit and vinegar." It's totally fine to have a large personality; just make sure you're tempered with politeness and civility.

Olives

Did you know that olives are a symbol for peace and friendship? This is where the expression "hand an olive branch" comes from, and nothing could be more impressive than thinking about mending relationships or creating new ones than when you add olives to a recipe. I also like that many olives are "pitted," which means the pit has been taken out, and what could be better than knowing you no longer have a "pit in your stomach," aka a worry or secret? If something has been bothering you, perhaps adding olives, whether pitted or not, can prompt you to remove the cause. Only you know if that means repairing a broken relationship, telling a secret in a safe way, or getting something off your chest. Like the dove, an olive branch is also a symbol of hope. Everyone needs hope. When you add olives to a recipe, take a mindful moment to name one or two things you are looking forward to and do your best to ensure that these things take place.

Finally, in some cultures, people plant an olive tree in memory of those who've passed. If you have a loved one you've lost, each olive can be a tiny moment of memory and fill your heart and perhaps the "pit" that was left behind.

Clear Your Plate

Now that you have the tools to create a cooking session based on the ingredients you choose, you have the complete tools to use cooking as therapy right in your own kitchen at any time you choose and for a complete set of challenges you're facing, issues you'd like to tackle, and choices you may want to entertain.

I'm so excited for you, as I know the journey you're about to embark on will be truly life-changing and you will be able to explore, evaluate, and elevate your mood, behaviors, and relationships with others as well as yourself. Plus you will never look at meal prep and food the same way, as you will always pull out the skills and tools you've learned at any time you feel the need. It's been so wonderful to share these tools with you, and it gives me great pleasure to say that after any cooking therapy session, it is the one time I will suggest that you "eat your feelings!" Enjoy, salud, bon appétit!

Conclusion: Check, Please

I hope you've found the lessons and sessions in this book helpful. More importantly, I hope you will use this book as a template and road map to visit all of the areas and situations in your life, even the ones that may not be mentioned in the book. Cooking therapy can add a dimension to your life every single day with every single meal or snack you prepare. Don't forget to use it for even the simplest moments. As you know by now, even a cracker with peanut butter can signify going crackers and nuts, something we should all do every day!

Remember that one bonus of cooking therapy is that you can ponder, revisit, and process the sessions at any time. Even if you don't redo a session, you can always revisit the steps and/or the to-go box.

With cooking as your therapy, you can create calm, infuse confidence, create self-acceptance, survive sadness, communicate better, make a change, and be heard. And cooking therapy is here for you to explore for just a few minutes or several hours. As with any other new skill, the more you practice, the more you will become proficient at recognizing negative self-talk, honestly evaluating feelings and behaviors, and changing styles and patterns if you so choose. At the very least, cooking therapy sessions will provide you with a disconnect from technology and a connection to yourself, a fresh way to evaluate what's positive and negative in your life and relationships, and a fun and creative opportunity to feel empowered. Remind yourself that there are no failures, only successful journeys.

Thank you for letting me come on this journey with you into your kitchens and into your hearts and minds.

Thanks for coming in, and I'll see you next week, or tomorrow, or whenever it works for you!

Warmly,
Debra Borden, your Sous Therapist™

Acknowledgments

First, I must thank my husband, David, for putting up with my writing alter ego, a scary, deranged monster who emerges when interrupted. Think large, bulging eyes, green face, smoke shooting out of the ears and nose, mouth screaming, "NOT NOW! I'M WRITING!" I wish this were an exaggeration. Honey, thank you for understanding, I love you, and I'm back. At least till the next book.

Next, thank you to my children, Erika and David, who I love to infinity and beyond, because nothing would be worthwhile doing or having without them in my life. Everything always is about the joy of them. I have the best kids. Not better than yours, I know. But ... well ... I kind of think maybe ... okay, fine, we'll leave it at that.

To my daughter-in-law Jamie, you are everything I could have hoped for and I love you to pieces.

There are two little princesses in my life named Dani Blake and Joey Gray. It's like having a pair of glowing Tinker Bells in my heart at all times. Their lights are so bright inside me and are everlasting and never dim. I miss them constantly, and sometimes I pretend air-kiss them on their cheeks and bellies as if they were here with me. That sounds weird, so don't tell anyone I said that.

To my amazing editor, Laura Apperson (I'm not sure who found who, but it was serendipity and symphony all at once)—mostly because of your talent, focus, and editing skills that deserve nothing less than a Kennedy Center

Honor. Just one thing: I now need therapy because I have an anxiety attack whenever I hear the phrase "Please expand." Thank you so much, Laura, for loving *Cooking as Therapy* from the beginning and guiding me to an end product that is really a collaboration I know we're both proud of. Many thanks to everyone at Alcove Press, including Thaisheemarie Fantauzzi Pérez, Dulce Botello, Mikaela Bender, Megan Matti, Stephanie Manova, and Rebecca Nelson, who all had a hand or maybe two in making *Cooking As Therapy* the beautiful book it has become.

To my equally delightful agent, Lindsey Smith of Spielburg Literary. You are a skilled engineer and excellent advocate, and equally impressive, you do it all while being a truly warm and nice person. What a joy to work with you! Sending fiction shortly...

To Stephanie and Marina Mulac, of 3 Wishes Studio, there is no other way to put this: You saved the existence of this book by convincing me not to quit, and you have been with me throughout this wonderful, amazing, and sometimes daunting journey and have believed in me and *Cooking As Therapy* from the beginning. Plus you are the only ones who tell me "You look great" when I do a video with a cold and bad hair. You are truly masters at what you do, and I am so grateful, and I love you for all that you do with both skill and joy.

To Julie Taylor, master of the proposal. Thank you for helping me get the *Cooking as Therapy* proposal into the kind of shape it needed to be so that others could see the book's worth and potential. I am forever grateful for your skill and collaboration.

Big hugs and thanks to my mainstays, the ones who are always there even when geography interferes: Jayne and Robin and my Jersey girls Terry, Rhonda, Debbie,

Barb, and Lynne. And to Laura, Lisa, Aric, Jayden, Rylen, Chelsea, Jeff, Carly, Matt, Leslee, Gene, Shelly Bruce, Lindsay, Sonny, and all the Buraks—family is everything, and I'm so lucky to have so many of you in my corner. I think about you often when writing but promise to keep you out of the novels.

And to my extended "tree branches," who support me always—you know who you are—from New Jersey, New York, Maryland, Georgia, and Florida, to Robin and Jack and my old and new friends at CHCC, Noyac, and SACC, thank you so much for your faith in me, for reading my novels, and for laughing at my essays. It means so much to think I've touched even one of you now and then. But mostly, thank you for your friendship.

Finally, endless hugs to the community of writers, foodies, chefs, social workers, and mental health professionals. When we support each other, the magic happens and we all grow exponentially, but you know that.

Resources

Resources When Feeling Stressed, Anxious, or Panicked

"Amygdala Hijack: When Emotion Takes Over": https://www.healthline.com/health/stress/amygdala-hijack

- Use this website to learn more about the physical causes of anxiety.

Creativity Reduces Stress: https://diversushealth.org /mental-health-blog/the-mental-health-benefits-of-creativity/

- Discover more about the ways creativity reduces stress and how you can incorporate it into your life.

Generalized Anxiety Disorder: https://www.nimh.nih .gov/health/publications/generalized-anxiety-disorder -gad

- For information on the clinical diagnosis of GAD, click this link to learn about the signs and symptoms.

Panic Attacks: https://www.nimh.nih.gov/health /publications/panic-disorder-when-fear-overwhelms

- How to recognize a panic attack and seek help for relief.

Amygdala Hijack: https://psychcentral.com/health
/amygdala-hijack#about-amygdala-hijack

- Extensive information on what happens in the brain
  to create anxiety and panic.

Sunshine Guilt: https://www.huffpost.com/entry
/sunshine-guilt-anxiety_l_6670879be4b08889dbe5d6e1

- If you feel guilty staying home when it's sunny
  outside, learn more about this little-known condition
  that affects many other people.

Resources When Experiencing Sadness or Depression

Depression Hotline USA: Dial 988. This call site is
manned 24/7.

Beck's Depression Inventory: https://www.ismanet.org
/doctoryourspirit/pdfs/Beck-Depression-Inventory-BDI.pdf

- A standardized test and/or self-test for features of
  and propensity for depression.

Resource When Addressing Eating Disorders

Renfrew Center: https://renfrewcenter.com/locations/

- Learn about eating disorders and where to seek help.

Cooking Therapy in Facilities and Treatment Centers and Within Organizations

Below is a list of mental health, substance abuse, and physical healing centers that are already incorporating cooking therapy into their programs.

Northeast Georgia/Lifepoint Cooking Therapy Room: https://nowhabersham.com/nghs-and-lifepoint -rehabilitation-to-build-new-inpatient-rehabilitation -facility/

Beachside Rehabs Culinary Healing: https://www .beachsiderehab.com/blog/culinary-healing-nourishing -your-body-and-mind/

Cirque Lodge Therapeutic Cooking: https://www .cirquelodge.com/treatment/experiential-therapy/cooking /#:~:text=Nourishing%20the%20Body%2C%20Mind%2C%20 and%20Soul%20at%20Cirque%20Lodge&text=On%20a%20 deeper%20level%2C%20it,out%20today%20to%20learn%20 more

Recovery Centers of America: https://www.youtube.com /watch?v=hyFVQZYbpgo

Alta Loma Transformational Services/Lionrock cooking therapy to aid recovery: https://www.altaloma.com /virtual-cooking-classes/

TerraBella Senior Living: https://www .terrabellaseniorliving.com/senior-living-blog/the -therapeutic-benefits-of-cooking-as-you-age/#:~:text =Engaging%20in%20culinary%20activities%20 can,older%20adults%20in%20numerous%20ways

Auburn Hill Senior Living: https://auburnhillliving.com/the-therapeutic-benefits-of-cooking-for-seniors/

Signal Mountain Assisted Living: https://signalmountainliving.com/blog/cooking-a-fun-and-therapeutic-activity-in-independent-living-apartments

The Chicago School: https://www.thechicagoschool.edu/insight/from-the-magazine/michael-kocet-culinary-therapy/

Finding a Culinary Therapist

Psychology Today: www.psychologytoday.com

- The number of therapists beginning to incorporate cooking therapy is growing! You can begin your search by visiting this website.

Bibliography

Allen, M. (n.d.). *America's ten favorite hobbies revealed: Our ten favorite ways to spend free time.* https://tools.e-exercises.com /doku.php?id=en:ecrit:articles-en:article_archive:america_s _favorite_hobbies_revealed:our_ten_favorite_ways_to_spend _free_time

Bashir, U. (2023, December 8). *Most popular hobbies & activities in the U.S. 2023.* Statista. https://www.statista.com/forecasts/997050/ most-popular-hobbies-and-activities-in-the-us

Brennan, D. (2021). *What to know about systematic desensitization.* WebMD. https://www.webmd.com/anxiety-panic/what-to-know -systematic-desensitization-therapy

Burnett, J. (2017, May 9). *Take a page out of Steve Jobs' book and switch to walking meetings.* Ladders. https://www.theladders.com /p/20506/steve-jobs-walking-meetings

Carlin, G. (Writer) & Urbisci, R. (Director). (1996). *George Carlin: George's best stuff* [Film]. MPI Home Video.

Clarke, J. (2024, January 12). *How gestalt therapy works.* https://www .verywellmind.com/what-is-gestalt-therapy-4584583#:~:text =Self%2DAwareness,-During%20gestalt%20therapy&text =Experiential%20exercise%20refers%20to%20 therapeutic,Awareness%20in%20itself%20is%20healing.%22

Cleveland Clinic. (2022, December 6). *Why giving is good for your health.* https://health.clevelandclinic.org/why-giving-is-good-for -your-health

Conner, T. S., DeYoung, C. G., & Silvia, P. J. (2018). Everyday creative activity as a path to flourishing. *The Journal of Positive*

Psychology, 13(2), 181–189. https://doi.org/10.1080/17439760.2016
.1257049

Cooking helped Bath woman with cancer through "darkest days."
(2024, August 19). BBC. https://www.bbc.com/news/articles/
cy793zz0l5io

Cue, D. (2017, April 25). Fill my cracks with gold. *The Coffeelicious.*
https://medium.com/the-coffeelicious/fill-my-cracks-with-gold
-375f86f8b900

Farmer, N., Touchton-Leonard, K., & Ross, A. (2018). Psychosocial
benefits of cooking interventions: A systematic review. *Health
Education & Behavior, 45*(2), 167–180. https://doi.org/10.1177
/1090198117736352

Friedlander, J. (2020, March 23). Perspective | How cooking became
the perfect recipe for my spiraling anxiety." *The Washington Post.*
https://www.washingtonpost.com/health/how-cooking-became
-the-perfect-recipe-for-my-spiralling-anxiety/2020/03/20
/a56d068a-4832-11ea-ab15-b5df3261b710_story.html

Gallary, C. (2015, April 16). *Can you really cook salmon in a dishwasher?* The Kitchn. https://www.thekitchn.com/can-you-really
-cook-salmon-in-a-dishwasher-putting-tips-to-the-test-in-the
-kitchn-218048

Goodwin, R. D., Dierker, L. C., Wu, M., Galea, S., Hoven, C. W., &
Weinberger, A. H. (2022). Trends in U.S. depression prevalence
from 2015 to 2020: The widening treatment gap. *American
Journal of Preventive Medicine, 63*(5), 726–733. https://doi.org/10
.1016/j.amepre.2022.05.014

Haidt, J. (2024). *The anxious generation: How the great rewiring of
childhood is causing an epidemic of mental illness.* Penguin.

Hamm, K. (2023, March 10). Study finds parents' phone use in front of
their kids can harm emotional intelligence. *The Current.* https://
news.ucsb.edu/2023/020867/screen-time-concerns

Horstman, E. (2024, August 6). *How "micro-moments" of mindfulness can help you find calm in the midst of chaos.* Camille

Styles. https://camillestyles.com/wellness/how-to-be-more
-mindful/

How cooking and connecting fully with food brings emotional,
mental and physical benefits—interviews. (2024, July 25). *South
China Morning Post.* https://www.scmp.com/lifestyle/100-top
-tables/article/3271784/how-cooking-and-connecting-fully-food
-brings-emotional-mental-and-physical-benefits-interviews

Ihsan, S. L. A. (2024, April 1). This home-based cook wants to help
postpartum mothers recover with healthy food. *The Star.* https://
www.thestar.com.my/lifestyle/family/2024/04/01/this-home
-based-cook-wants-to-help-postpartum-mothers-recover-with
-healthy-food

Johnson, C. (1955). *Harold and the purple crayon.* Harper and Brothers.

Kaimal, G. (2024, June 20). *Making art is a uniquely human act, and one
that provides a wellspring of health benefits.* The Conversation.
https://theconversation.com/making-art-is-a-uniquely-human-act
-and-one-that-provides-a-wellspring-of-health-benefits-219091

Kalaichandran, A. (2018, May 22). The doctor is cooking. *The New
York Times.* https://www.nytimes.com/2018/05/22/well/eat
/doctors-kitchen-cooking-food-patients-nutrition.html

Kitchen therapy: Cooking up mental well-being. (n.d.). *Psychology
Today.* https://www.psychologytoday.com/us/blog/minding-the-
body/201505/kitchen-therapy-cooking-mental-well-being

Kraut, M. (2023). *Children and grooming / online predators.* Child
Crime Prevention & Safety Center. https://childsafety
.losangelescriminallawyer.pro/children-and-grooming-online
-predators.html

LaGuardia, G. (2024, April 15). *Culinary healing: Nourishing your
body and mind.* Beachside Rehab. https://www.beachsiderehab
.com/blog/culinary-healing-nourishing-your-body-and-mind/

Lee, L. (2019, June 28). *Therapists use cooking to stir up better mental
health.* CNN. https://www.cnn.com/2019/06/28/health/sw
-culinary-arts-therapy-cooking/index.html

Locker, M. (2022, August 1). The emotional benefits of cooking. *Southern Living.* https://www.southernliving.com/healthy-living/mind-body/cooking-therapy-mental-health

Mayo Clinic Staff. (2023, September 22). *Stress relief from laughter? It's no joke.* Mayo Clinic. https://www.mayoclinic.org/healthy-lifestyle/stress-management/in-depth/stress-relief/art-20044456

MIT Media Lab Tangible Media Group. (n.d.). *Design of haptic interfaces for psychotherapy.* Massachusetts Institute of Technology, School of Architecture and Planning. Retrieved December 20, 2024, from https://tangible.media.mit.edu/project/psychohaptics/

NGHS and Lifepoint Rehabilitation to build new inpatient rehab facility. (2023, April 3). Now Habersham. https://nowhabersham.com/nghs-and-lifepoint-rehabilitation-to-build-new-inpatient-rehabilitation-facility/

Pacheco, I. (2012, January 9). *The stages of change (Prochaska & DiClemente).* Social Work Tech. https://socialworktech.com/2012/01/09/stages-of-change-prochaska-diclemente/

Schonfeld, A. (2023). Cyberbullying and adolescent suicide. *The Journal of the American Academy of Psychiatry and the Law, 51*(1), 112–119. https://doi.org/10.29158/JAAPL.220078-22

Shah, S. (2024, June 17). U.S. surgeon general wants a warning label for social media. *TIME.* https://time.com/6989369/us-surgeon-general-warning-label-social-media/

Straus, M. B. (2023). *No-talk therapy for children and adolescents.* W. W. Norton.

Thomson, J. R. (2017, April 17). *How something called 'culinary arts therapy' can change your life.* HuffPost. https://www.huffpost.com/entry/culinary-arts-therapy_n_58ee79c1e4b0bb9638e0e02b

Turner, V. S. (2016, January 5). The strain of always being on call. *Scientific American.* https://www.scientificamerican.com/article/the-strain-of-always-being-on-call/

Wampold, B. E. (2015). How important are the common factors in psychotherapy? an update. *World Psychiatry, 14*(3), 270–277. https://doi.org/10.1002/wps.20238

Weilkiens, T. (2007). *General system theory—an overview.* ScienceDirect. https://www.sciencedirect.com/topics/computer-science /general-system-theory

Whalen, J. (2014, December 8). A road to mental health through the kitchen. *Wall Street Journal.* https://www.wsj.com/articles/a-road -to-mental-health-through-the-kitchen-1418059204.

Zilcha-Mano, S., Solomonov, N., Chui, H., McCarthy, K. S., Barrett, M. S., & Barber, J. P. (2015). Therapist-reported alliance: Is it really a predictor of outcome? *Journal of Counseling Psychology, 62*(4), 568–578. https://doi.org/10.1037/cou0000106

Index

01 14

√ √